CALL TO POST

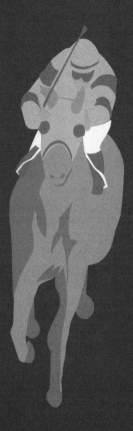

Winning Kentucky Recipes

Additional copies may be obtained at the cost of $18.95 each book, plus $3.50 postage and handling per order. Kentucky residents add $1.14 sales tax, each book.

Send to:

Call To Post
635 Iron Works Pike
Lexington, Kentucky 40511
(606) 293-6579

ISBN Number 0-9656246-1-7

First Printing   March 1997   10,000 copies

Printed in the USA by
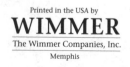
WIMMER
The Wimmer Companies, Inc.
Memphis

TABLE OF CONTENTS

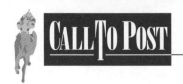

INTRODUCTION

Two centuries ago Daniel Boone walked across the Cumberland Gap into Kentucky and opened up the beautiful, rolling, limestone-rich land that has gone on to foster the finest Thoroughbred horse farms in the world. Rich in tradition, the Bluegrass region of central Kentucky is home to standardbreds and saddlebreds as well as Thoroughbreds, making Lexington the undisputed horse capital of the world. Illustrious stallions Lexington and Man o' War established the Bluegrass as the center of Thoroughbred breeding around the turn of the century. Since that time, people from all parts of the world have come to Kentucky to pursue the dream of owning a winner of the Kentucky Derby, England's Epsom Derby or France's Arc de Triomphe.

For decades the masters of Kentucky's horse farms have played hosts to notable figures from the capitals and playgrounds of the world, entertaining royalty, business magnates and sportsmen. Several times a year these luminaries come to Lexington to indulge their passion for horses. Bluegrass hosts fete their visitors with garden parties, elegant dinners, cocktail buffets, picnics and brunches. Some of the most prominent farms are pictured and described in **CALL TO POST**.

CALL TO POST captures the recipes prepared by renowned Bluegrass chefs, caterers, hosts and hostesses to entertain these guests. As diverse as horsemen themselves, the cookbook offers everything from updated favorites and quick, tasty daily fare to creative ideas for hors d'oeuvres, elegant dishes and innovative new creations.

Proceeds from **CALL TO POST** benefit the Lexington Hearing and Speech Center in Lexington, Kentucky. Since 1960, the Center's sole mission has been to bring the joy of communication to those it serves. With its beginnings deeply rooted in preschool programming for hearing-impaired children, the Center is now a premier agency that offers comprehensive clinical and educational services for individuals with hearing and speech problems.

It is our earnest wish that you enjoy both preparing and eating the food from the recipes on the pages of this Bluegrass classic. Bon appétit.

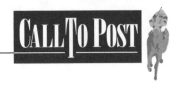

Beth Clifton—Editor
Bob May—Fund Raising Chairman

CHAPTER EDITORS

Harriet Bradley
Pattie Broadbent
Elizabeth Dupree
Mary Wis Estes

Linda Gaitskill
Karen Hollins
Marjorie Holzfeind
Betsy Lankford
Maggie Metcalf

Beth Poulton
Robin Snowden
Meg Sprow
Holly Van Dissel

FRIENDS OF COOKBOOK

Ann Asbury
Web Cowden
Doug Dean
Mary Wis Estes
Edith Frankel

Juanice Gillespie
William Green
Stan Kerrick
Bernadette Mattox
John Milward

Carol Nicholas
Anne Rogers
Michael Scanlon
Marie Sprague
Barbara Young

RECIPE CONTRIBUTORS

Jenny Dulworth Albert
Anna Jean Altizer
Karen Anderson
Holly Arnold
Ann Asbury
Julia Ashman
Diane Avare
Melinda Bates
Debi Bathrick
Ann Banks
Beth Barr
Mary Berge
Leslie Berkley
Mary Bolt

Tricia Boone
Peggy Borders
John Bryant
Kim Bunch
Bettye Burns
Peggy Cains
Julie Cashman
Mary Cherrey
Kip Clifton
Debbie Coleman
Sally Corrigan
Kathy Courtney
Web Cowden
Susan Crissy

Joni Dalton
Doug Dean
Susan Douglass
Phil Dunn
Laura Edwards
Page Edwards
Page Estes
Kathy Feinberg
Gail Figgs
Edith Frankel
Grayce Franks
Elizabeth Freeman
Mary H. Gabbert
Jo Gangthrop

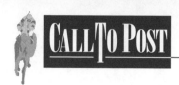
Juanice Gillespie
Julie Anne Grady
William Green
Sylvia Griffin
Mary Donna Hadden
Julia Hall
Wendy Haney
Charline Hardwick
Jessica Harrison
Suzy Hayes
Joan Henning
Tom Holzfeind
Francie Houlihan
Carol Hustedde
Marilyn Hynson
Del Kelly
Martha Kerrick
Melodye Kinkead
Mary Kittinger
Denise Koenig
Lee Lamonica
Alana Leffler
Wendy Lewis
Janice MacNeil
Leann W. Marcum
Chris Martin
Susan Mastin
Ginny May
Martie Mayer

Katherine McCarty
Libby McCarty
Louise McDermott
Tracy McKinley
Lisa Miller
Luanne Milward
Bunnie Mologne
Keely Mooney
Lola Murray
Carol Nicholas
Jane Allen Offutt
Becky Ogle
Missy O'Mera
Lucy Owen
Marianne Patterson
Martha Poulton
Peggy Queen
Mary Ann Rafferty
Elizabeth Remmers
Maria Roach
Elizabeth Robbins
Jessica Robbins
Anne Rogers
Marilyn Rosenwein
Nancy Roszell
Missy Scanlon
E. Schobel
Sally Schreiber
Bobby Scrivner

Karen Sheetz
Nancy Williamson
   Simpson
Marilyn Smith
Betty Snowden
Phaedra Spradlin
Marie Sprague
Jean Stafford
Dot Ewing Stagich
Shannon Stephens
Julia Stevens
Bill Straus
Lisa Summerlin
Kathleen Sweeney
Shannon Totty
Sue Ann Truitt
Chef Edward Valente
Charlene Vanderbrink
Patty Walter
Beth Weisenberger
Dorcas Wiedemann
Martha Wiedemann
Teresa Wilhite
Sallie Wilkinson
Amy Williams
Bookie Wilson
Sherri Wolf
Barbara Young

ARTISTS

Cover Art   Anne Melnyk
Divider Art   Cary Tsamas

Appetizers & Beverages

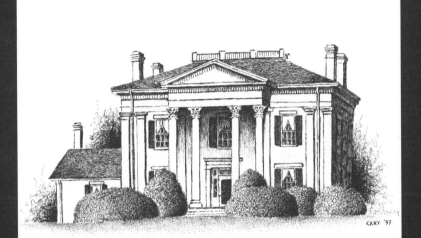

Payson Stud, on the legendary Paris Pike, was established by Virginia Kraft Payson and her late husband, Charles Shipman Payson, in 1980. Its 300-plus acres, originally parts of Greentree and Duntreath Farms, are currently home to multiple Champion and 1992 European Horse of the Year, St. Jovite, and his dam, Northern Sunset (IRE), 1995 Broodmare of the Year. Northern Sunset has also produced the millionaires, L'Carriere and Salem Drive, as well as the multiple Graded Stakes winner, Lac Ouimet. All were homebreds, carrying the farm's distinctive silks, consisting of a blue square on a white background.

Payson Stud

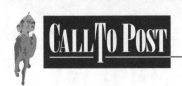

Appetizers & Beverages

Appetizers

Beverages

SPICY BLACK BEAN AND CORN SALSA

Combine bell peppers, jalapeño peppers, beans, corn, cilantro, green onion, red onion, lime juice, oil, cumin and salt in large container. Season with black pepper. Chill, covered, for at least 2 hours or overnight. Add tomatoes just before serving. Serve with toasted pita triangles or blue and white corn chips.

Makes 7 to 8 cups.

1   green bell pepper, diced
1   red bell pepper, diced
2   jalapeño peppers, chopped
1   pound cooked black beans
1   pound fresh or frozen corn
⅓   cup chopped fresh cilantro
¼   cup chopped green onion
¼   cup chopped red onion
⅓   cup fresh lime juice
3   tablespoons vegetable oil
1   tablespoon ground cumin
1   teaspoon salt
    Freshly ground black pepper
    to taste
½   cup chopped ripe tomatoes,
    drained

CAVIAR PIE

Pie can be prepared in advance. Cover loosely with plastic wrap and store in refrigerator until ready to serve.

Blend cream and sour cream until smooth. Spread evenly in decorative 8- or 9-inch pie plate. Peel eggs, cut in halves and remove yolks. Separately chop whites and yolks. Mound black caviar on center of cream cheese layer. In order listed, surround caviar with ring of egg yolk, scallions, red caviar, egg whites and parsley. Serve with crackers or party rye slices.

Serves 12 to 16.

1   8-ounce package cream
    cheese, softened
3   tablespoons low-fat sour
    cream
4   hard-cooked eggs
1   ounce black caviar, drained
    on paper towel
1   ounce red caviar, drained on
    paper towel
4   or 5 scallions (green portion
    only), minced
½   cup minced fresh parsley

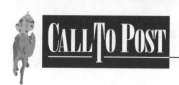

SOUTH OF THE BORDER DIP

BEANS
1 15-ounce can or 2 cups cooked
black beans
4½ cups cold water
1 tablespoon minced garlic
1 small yellow onion, chopped
1½ teaspoons cumin seed
1 teaspoon dried marjoram
1 bay leaf
1 teaspoon salt

TORTILLA WEDGES
4 6-inch corn tortillas
2 tablespoons cold water
½ teaspoon salt
⅛ teaspoon cayenne pepper

VEGETABLES
1 large red bell pepper
1 large yellow bell pepper
3 large ripe tomatoes, cored and
diced
4 green onions, finely chopped
½ avocado, peeled, seeded and
diced
¼ cup chopped fresh cilantro
2 tablespoons fresh lime juice
2 tablespoons finely grated
lime zest
2 teaspoons vinegar
¼ teaspoon salt
¼ teaspoon freshly ground red
pepper
2 small jalapeño peppers,
cored, seeded and chopped
¼ cup (1 ounce) crumbled goat
cheese
Finely grated lime zest for
garnish
Fresh cilantro sprigs for
garnish

Combine beans, water, garlic, onion, cumin, marjoram and bay leaf in large saucepan. Bring to a boil, reduce heat to low and simmer for 40 minutes. Stir in salt and continue cooking for about 15 minutes or until very soft. Remove from heat and drain, reserving liquid. Discard bay leaf. Place ½ of bean mixture and ⅓ cup of reserved liquid in food processor, purée until smooth and add to remaining bean mixture. Bean mixture can be prepared in advance and stored overnight in refrigerator.

Cut tortillas into quarters. Combine cold water, salt and cayenne. Brush lightly on both sides of tortilla quarters and place on baking sheets. Bake at 350° for 12 minutes or until crisp. Wedges can be prepared in advance and stored in airtight container overnight.

Roast red and yellow peppers. Let stand until cool, peel, dice and set aside. Combine tomatoes, green onion, avocado, cilantro, lime juice, 2 tablespoons lime zest, vinegar, salt and red pepper. In deep 1½-quart bowl, layer ½ of bean mixture, bell peppers, jalapeño peppers, tomato mixture and goat cheese; repeat layers and garnish with lime zest and cilantro. Serve with warm tortilla wedges or purchased tortilla chips.

Serves 8.

HOT CHIPOTLE SALSA

Combine tomatoes, cilantro, lime juice, chipotle chilies and cumin. Season with salt and black pepper. Serve on hamburgers, in chili or with tortilla chips. **Note:** Chipotle chilies in adobo sauce are available at specialty foods stores and some supermarkets.

Makes 4 cups.

3 to 4 cups chopped tomatoes
¾ cup chopped fresh cilantro
¼ cup fresh lime juice
1½ tablespoons chopped canned chipotle chilies in adobo sauce
1½ teaspoons ground cumin
Salt and black pepper to taste

MEXICAN SALAD DIP

Combine tomatoes, olives, chilies and onions. Blend oil, vinegar and salt together. Pour liquid over vegetables and mix thoroughly. Serve with chips.

Makes 2 cups.

2 medium-ripe tomatoes, finely chopped
1 4-ounce can black olives, chopped
1 4-ounce can green chilies, chopped
3 or 4 green onions, chopped
3 tablespoons olive oil
½ tablespoon red wine vinegar
1 teaspoon garlic salt

CHUTNEY CHEESE BALL

Combine butter, Cheddar cheese and cream cheese. Shape into a ball and chill for several hours. Roll cheese ball in onion, bacon and chutney, covering well. Serve with crackers.

Makes 2½ cups.

½ cup butter, softened
1 cup (4 ounces) grated Cheddar cheese
1 8-ounce package cream cheese, softened
1 bunch green onions, chopped
½ pound bacon, cooked and crumbled
1 9-ounce jar chutney

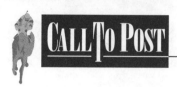

CRANBERRY-TOPPED BRIE

Cheese can be heated in microwave oven.

½ cup canned cranberry-orange
    sauce
2 tablespoons brown sugar
¼ cup chopped pecans
1 tablespoon brandy
1 round Brie cheese

Combine cranberry-orange sauce, brown sugar, pecans and brandy. Cut circle from top of cheese rind, leaving ¼-inch rim around edge. Place in ovenproof dish. Spoon cranberry mixture on exposed cheese. Bake at 500° for 5 to 8 minutes or until cheese is thoroughly heated.

Serves 6 to 8.

GOAT CHEESE AND BROCCOLI SPREAD

2 cups broccoli flowerets
1 8-ounce package goat cheese,
   softened
2 3-ounce packages cream
   cheese, softened
   Salt and black pepper to taste
   Toasted pita wedges
   Sun-dried tomatoes for
   garnish

Blanch broccoli by submerging in boiling water for a few minutes, then plunging in ice water, or microwave cook for 5 minutes. Cool slightly. Combine goat cheese and cream cheese in food processor, mixing until smooth. Season with salt and black pepper. Add broccoli and process just until blended. Spread mixture on wedges and garnish with tomatoes.

Makes 3 cups.

DILL SHRIMP

1½ cups mayonnaise
½   cup sour cream
⅓   cup fresh lemon juice
¼   cup sugar
¼   teaspoon salt
2   tablespoons dill weed
1   large red onion, thinly sliced
2   pounds shrimp, cooked,
    peeled and deveined

A day in advance of serving, blend mayonnaise, sour cream, lemon juice, sugar, salt and dill weed. Stir in onion and shrimp. Chill overnight.

Serves 10 to 12.

TOMATO CHEESE SPREAD

Beat cream cheese until smooth. Add tomatoes, green onion, pecans, salt and Worcestershire sauce, mixing thoroughly. Serve with crackers.

Makes 1½ cups.

1	8-ounce package cream cheese, softened
¼	cup oil-packed sun-dried tomatoes, chopped and drained
4	green onions, chopped
¼	cup chopped pecans
½	teaspoon salt
	Worcestershire sauce to taste

SHRIMP DIP

Combine mayonnaise, sour cream, ketchup, onion, sherry, cayenne pepper and Worcestershire sauce. Stir in shrimp. Chill. Serve with crackers or toasted French bread rounds.

Makes 2½ cups.

¾	cup mayonnaise
¾	cup sour cream
2	tablespoons ketchup
2	tablespoons minced fresh onion
2	tablespoons dry sherry
¼	teaspoon cayenne pepper
1½	teaspoons Worcestershire sauce
1¼	pounds shrimp, cooked, peeled, deveined and coarsely chopped

STEAK FINGERS

Partially freeze steak to make slicing easier.

Cut steak on diagonal into thin slices. Roll up, securing with wooden picks. Combine oil, soy sauce, honey, vinegar, garlic powder, ginger, mustard and onion powder, blending well. Marinate beef rolls in sauce, turning to coat on all sides. Remove rolls from sauce and grill over hot coals or heat source for 5 minutes, turn and grill on second side for 5 minutes.

Serves 8 to 10.

2	pounds flank steak
¾	cup vegetable oil
½	cup soy sauce
2	tablespoons honey
2	tablespoons cider vinegar
1	teaspoon garlic powder
1	teaspoon grated fresh ginger
⅛	teaspoon dry mustard
1	teaspoon onion powder

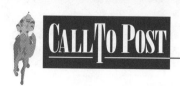

CAJUN MARINATED SHRIMP WITH RÉMOULADE SAUCE

SHRIMP
⅓ cup salt
¼ cup black pepper
¼ cup garlic powder
2 tablespoons cayenne pepper
3 tablespoons onion powder
2 tablespoons oregano
¼ cup paprika
2 tablespoons dried thyme
3 pounds (30-count per pound) medium shrimp, peeled and deveined

Combine salt, black pepper, garlic powder, cayenne pepper, onion powder, oregano, paprika and thyme, mixing thoroughly. Sprinkle mixture over shrimp, tossing to coat thoroughly. Sauté shrimp in large skillet, cooking just until done. Cool to room temperature and serve with Rémoulade Sauce.

Serves 8 to 10.

RÉMOULADE SAUCE
¼ cup Creole mustard
½ cup prepared mustard
½ cup white vinegar
½ cup ketchup
3 eggs, at room temperature
Juice of 1 lemon
1 cup minced green onion
1 cup finely chopped celery
1 cup finely chopped parsley
2 cloves garlic, minced
1 teaspoon salt
1 teaspoon cayenne pepper
2 tablespoons paprika
Dash of hot pepper sauce
1⅓ cups vegetable oil

Combine Creole mustard, prepared mustard, vinegar, ketchup, eggs, lemon juice, green onion, celery, parsley, garlic, salt, cayenne pepper, paprika and hot pepper sauce in blender. Mix until well blended. Gradually add oil in steady stream to mustard mixture, mixing until thickened to mayonnaise consistency. Chill.

Makes 6 cups.

CRAB QUESADILLAS

Grilled chicken can be substituted for crab.

Combine cheese, cilantro, scallions, garlic, jalapeño pepper, cumin, salt and black pepper, mixing well. Pour small amount of oil in large skillet over medium heat. Place 2 tortillas in skillet. Spoon portion of cheese mixture on each. When cheese begins to melt, spoon portion of crab meat on 1 of tortillas. Flip other tortilla onto crab-covered tortilla and continue cooking, flipping once, until both sides are gold brown. Place on baking sheet and set aside. Repeat with remaining ingredients. Reheat tortillas at 400° for 5 minutes, turning once. Let stand for 2 minutes to allow cheese to become firm, then slice in 8 wedges. Spoon salsa and tomato on each wedge. Serve immediately.

Makes 64.

2   **cups (8 ounces) grated Monterey Jack cheese**
¼   **cup chopped fresh cilantro**
¼   **cup chopped scallions**
1   **clove garlic, minced**
1   **tablespoon minced jalapeño pepper**
1   **tablespoon cumin**
½   **teaspoon salt**
1   **teaspoon black pepper**
½   **cup olive oil**
1½   **cups crab meat**
8   **flour tortillas**
½   **cup salsa**
½   **cup diced tomato**

OYSTERS OVER TOAST

Cook bacon in skillet until crisp. Remove, drain on paper towel and set aside. Retaining about 2 tablespoons bacon drippings in skillet, add oysters with liquid and cook over medium heat until edges begin to curl. Stir in lemon juice. Serve oysters with sauce on toast, crumbling bacon over each serving.

Serves 6.

4   **slices bacon**
1   **pint oysters with liquid**
    Juice of 1 lemon
6   **slices bread, crisply toasted**

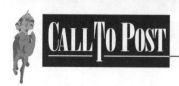

CAJUN CHICKEN BITES WITH APRICOT MUSTARD

Chicken can also be served as an entrée.

CHICKEN

5   chicken breast halves, bone and skin removed, cut in bite-sized pieces
2   tablespoons unsalted butter
2   tablespoons vegetable oil

Prepare apricot mustard and spice mix. Sprinkle spice mix on chicken and let stand for about 30 minutes. Sauté chicken in butter and oil in skillet over medium-high heat for about 5 minutes or just until done. Remove with slotted spoon and drain briefly on paper towel. Serve hot with apricot mustard.

APRICOT MUSTARD

1½   cups apricot preserves
¼   cup plus 2 tablespoons Creole or Dijon mustard

Combine preserves and mustard in small saucepan. Cook over low heat, stirring to mix, until preserves are melted and thoroughly blended with mustard. Set aside to cool.

CAJUN SPICE MIX

1   tablespoon garlic powder
1   teaspoon salt or to taste
2   teaspoons ground cayenne pepper
2   teaspoons freshly ground black pepper
1   teaspoon freshly ground white pepper
2   teaspoons dried thyme, finely crumbled

Combine garlic, salt, cayenne pepper, black pepper, white pepper and thyme in plastic bag or small bowl, shaking or stirring to mix well.

Serves 8 to 10.

CHICKEN SATÉ WITH PEANUT SAUCE

Prepare marinade and peanut sauce. Thread chicken pieces on skewers. Place in marinade and let stand at room temperature for at least 2 hours or in refrigerator overnight for more intense flavor. Prepare moderate charcoal fire in open grill or preheat broiler. Cook chicken, turning several times and basting with marinade, over medium-hot coals or under broiler for about 6 to 8 minutes or until crispy on outside but moist on inside. Sprinkle with lime zest and garnish with cilantro leaves. Serve with peanut sauce for dipping.

Combine brown sugar, curry powder, peanut butter, soy sauce, lime juice, garlic and crushed chilies in shallow dish.

Combine peanut butter, coconut milk, lemon juice, soy sauce, brown sugar or molasses, ginger, garlic and cayenne pepper in saucepan. Cook over medium heat, stirring constantly, for about 15 minutes or until sauce is consistency of whipping cream. Pour into food processor or blender and purée. Add broth and cream. Blend until smooth. Sauce can be made several hours in advance and stored in refrigerator until ready to use. Bring to room temperature before serving.

Makes 18.

CHICKEN
6   chicken breast halves, skin and bone removed, cut in strips ½-inch wide
    Grated lime zest for garnish
    Fresh cilantro sprigs for garnish

MARINADE
1   tablespoon light brown sugar
1   tablespoon curry powder
2   tablespoons crunchy peanut butter
½   cup low sodium soy sauce
½   cup fresh lime juice
2   garlic cloves, minced
    Crushed dried red chili peppers to taste

PEANUT SAUCE
⅔   cup crunchy peanut butter
1½ cups unsweetened coconut milk
¼   cup fresh lemon juice
2   tablespoons soy sauce
2   tablespoons brown sugar or molasses
1   teaspoon grated fresh ginger root
4   cloves garlic, minced
    Ground cayenne pepper to taste
¼   cup fresh chicken broth or canned low-sodium broth
¼   cup whipping cream

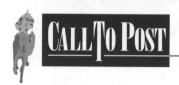

HAM BUNDLES

Appetizer can be assembled in advance and stored in refrigerator until ready to bake. Allow a few more minutes for heating.

1   cup butter
3   tablespoons prepared yellow mustard
3   tablespoons poppy seeds
1   onion, chopped
1   teaspoon Worcestershire sauce
2   cups (8 ounces) shredded Swiss cheese
3   packages prepared party rolls
1   pound ham, shaved or thinly sliced

Melt butter in skillet. Stir in mustard, poppy seeds, onion, Worcestershire sauce and cheese. Remove from heat and set aside. Keeping tops and bottoms intact, cut rolls in half horizontally. Place ham on bottom section, spread cheese mixture on top section, place sections and wrap in aluminum foil. Bake at 375° for about 10 minutes or until thoroughly heated. Cut into individual sandwiches and serve warm.

Makes 36.

ANTIPASTO-STUFFED PEASANT LOAF

2   small (16x2x1-inch) baguettes
¼   cup bottled olive paste or tapenade
1   4-ounce package mild goat cheese
¼   pound thinly sliced Genoa salami or smoked turkey
2   cups packed fresh arugula or spinach leaves
1   7-ounce jar roasted red peppers, drained, rinsed and blotted dry
1   14-ounce can whole artichoke hearts, drained, rinsed, blotted dry and chopped

Using serrated knife, horizontally cut top ⅓ from each baguette. Remove soft crumbs from top and bottom portions, leaving shells about ½ inch thick. Spread about 1 tablespoon olive paste or tapenade on inside of each bottom shell and spread evenly with goat cheese. Fold salami or turkey slices in halves and arrange in layer over cheese in each shell. Layer arugula or spinach on meat, add roasted peppers and top with artichoke hearts. Spread remaining olive paste or tapenade on inside of top shells. Fit top shells over bottom shells and press together, re-forming loaves. Wrap each tightly in aluminum foil. Chill for at least 3 hours or overnight. Cut each baguette diagonally into 12 slices and secure with wooden pick.

Makes 24.

VIETNAMESE PORK ROLL-UPS

Rolls can also be served as an entrée.

Combine pork, chestnuts, garlic, onion, soy sauce, vegetable oil, lemon juice, ginger, sugar, oil and salt, mixing thoroughly. Roll meat mixture into about 20 2-inch links. Sauté in skillet over medium heat until thoroughly cooked. Set aside to drain on paper towel and keep warm. Prepare dipping sauce. Prepare garnishes and place in small serving bowls. To assemble, place meat patty on lettuce leaf, sprinkle with garnishes, roll leaf to enclose and dip into sauce.

Combine soy sauce, lemon juice, water, garlic, sugar, oyster sauce, ginger and cayenne pepper in small saucepan. Bring to a boil, reduce heat and simmer for 5 minutes. Let stand until cool.

Makes 20.

FILLING
1½ pounds lean ground pork
6 water chestnuts, minced
1 large clove garlic, minced
1 green onion, minced
1 tablespoon soy sauce
2 teaspoons vegetable oil
1¼ teaspoons fresh lemon juice
½ teaspoon grated fresh ginger
¼ teaspoon sugar
¼ teaspoon hot chili oil
⅛ teaspoon salt
Boston or bibb lettuce leaves, washed and blotted dry

DIPPING SAUCE
½ cup soy sauce
¼ cup plus 1 tablespoon lemon juice
3 tablespoons water
2 cloves garlic, minced
2 teaspoons sugar
1 teaspoon oyster sauce
1 teaspoon grated fresh ginger
¼ teaspoon cayenne pepper

GARNISHES
½ cup chopped fresh cilantro
½ cup chopped green onion
½ cup chopped fresh mint

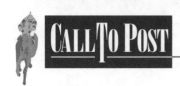

STUFFED CHERRY TOMATOES

1 6-ounce can crabmeat, drained
1 cup cooked shrimp, chopped
2 green onions, chopped
⅛ teaspoon red pepper
1 tablespoon fresh lemon juice
¼ cup mayonnaise
30 large cherry tomatoes
    Fresh parsley sprigs

Combine crabmeat, shrimp, green onion, red pepper, lemon juice and mayonnaise in food processor, mixing until smooth or blending by hand. Cut an x-shape on bottom of each tomato, cutting to within ½ inch of stem end. Remove pulp from tomato and invert on paper towel to drain. Spoon seafood mixture into each tomato and garnish with parsley sprig.

Makes 30.

CROSTINI AL POMODORO
(TOASTED BREAD WITH CHOPPED TOMATOES)
A great summer appetizer when tomatoes are fresh and plentiful.

TOMATO MIXTURE
3 ripe tomatoes, peeled, seeded and chopped
3 or 4 large cloves garlic, minced
¼ cup chopped fresh basil
    Salt and black pepper to taste
3 tablespoons olive oil

Combine tomatoes, garlic, basil, salt and black pepper. Add olive oil to moisten. Set aside or chill if not serving immediately.

BREAD
1 loaf Italian bread or French baguette
3 or 4 cloves garlic
¼ to ½ cup olive oil

Prepare tomato mixture. Cut bread diagonally into thin slices. Blend garlic and oil in food processor. Brush each side of bread with flavored oil. Place on baking sheet. Toast, turning once, at 350° until edges of bread begin to brown. Spoon tomato mixture on each slice.

Serves 10 to 12.

GORGONZOLA CROSTINI

6 breadsticks, cut in ¼-inch rounds
¼ cup butter, melted
1 4-ounce package Gorgonzola cheese
¼ cup butter, softened
1 cup chopped pecans

Brush breadstick slices with melted butter and place on baking sheet. Bake at 375° for 7 minutes. Combine cheese, softened butter and pecans, mixing well. Place 1 teaspoonful of cheese nut mixture on each bread slice. Bake for 10 minutes. Serve warm.

Makes 60.

SPINACH AND BACON PUFFS

1 17-ounce package frozen puff pastry
½ 10-ounce package frozen chopped spinach, thawed and well-drained
1 3-ounce package cream cheese, softened
1 tablespoon milk
2 tablespoons thinly sliced green onion
3 slices bacon, cooked and crumbled
2 tablespoons finely chopped pimento
1 egg, beaten
1 tablespoon water

Let pastry stand at room temperature for 20 minutes. While pastry thaws, prepare filling. Combine spinach, cream cheese, milk, green onion, bacon and pimento, mixing well. Blend egg and water in separate bowl. On lightly floured surface, roll each pastry sheet to form 15x12-inch rectangle. Cut each sheet in 3-inch squares. Spoon portion of spinach mixture in center of each square and brush edges with egg mixture. Fold pastry diagonally over filling to form triangle, press edges with fork tines to seal and place on ungreased baking sheet. Brush top of triangles with egg mixture. Bake at 425° for 12 to 15 minutes or until pastry is golden and filling is hot.

Makes 40.

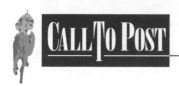

QUICK CALZONE

Very easy.

1	8-ounce can refrigerated French bread dough
¼	pound pepperoni, thinly sliced
1	cup (4 ounces) grated mozzarella cheese
¼	cup thinly sliced red bell pepper
1	egg yolk, beaten

Roll dough to form rectangle. Sprinkle pepperoni, cheese and bell pepper on dough. Beginning from longer edge, roll tightly, pinch seam to seal and place on baking sheet. Brush top with egg yolk. Bake, on bottom rack, at 350° for about 45 minutes or until golden brown. Cool slightly, slice and serve warm. **Note:** Other combinations can be used for filling, such as prosciutto ham, Cheddar cheese and broccoli.

Serves 6 to 8.

SMOKED SALMON PINWHEELS

1	8-ounce package cream cheese, softened
2	tablespoons fresh lemon juice
1	teaspoon hot pepper sauce
¼	cup chopped red onion
4	flour tortillas
¼	cup capers
½	pound thinly sliced smoked salmon
	Lemon slices for garnish
	Dill sprigs for garnish

Blend cream cheese, lemon juice and hot pepper sauce together until smooth. Spread evenly on tortillas. Sprinkle onion and capers on cream cheese and add layer of salmon slices. Roll each tortilla, jelly roll style, and place seam side down on plate. Chill, covered with plastic wrap, until firm. Cut rolls into pinwheel slices just before serving. Garnish with lemon slices and dill sprigs.

Makes 36 to 40.

OLD SOUTH CHEESE STRAWS

Combine 1 cup Cheddar cheese and ½ cup butter in food processor. Using steel blade, cream until smooth. Add 1⅓ cups flour, ¼ teaspoon salt and ¼ teaspoon cayenne pepper, processing until dough forms ball around blade. Remove and shape into ball. Repeat with remaining ingredients. Chill dough for 1 hour. Form straws and place on ungreased baking sheet. Bake at 275° for 20 to 25 minutes or until crispy.

Makes 48.

2   cups (8 ounces) grated extra-sharp Cheddar cheese
1   cup butter
2⅔   cups sifted all-purpose flour
½   teaspoon salt
½   teaspoon cayenne pepper

SPICY PECANS

Melt butter in large saucepan. Blend in Worcestershire sauce, ketchup and hot pepper sauce. Add pecans, stirring to coat thoroughly with sauce. Spread pecans evenly in 13x9x2-inch baking dish. Bake at 400° for 20 minutes, stirring frequently; avoid burning. Spoon pecans on paper towel and sprinkle with salt.

Makes 4 cups.

2   tablespoons butter
¼   cup Worcestershire sauce
1   tablespoon ketchup
4   dashes hot pepper sauce
4   cups pecan halves
     Salt

SMOOTHIE

A wonderful way to start your day!

Combine yogurt, banana, blueberries, strawberries, orange juice and vanilla in blender. Process until smooth. Serve in chilled glass with strawberry garnish.

Serves 6.

1   cup low-fat strawberry yogurt
1   ripe banana, frozen
1   cup fresh or frozen blueberries
1   cup fresh or frozen strawberries
1½   cups orange juice
¼   teaspoon vanilla
6   whole fresh strawberries

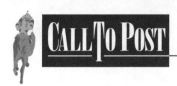

YUMMY SLUSHY PUNCH

1   3-ounce package strawberry
    or cherry gelatin
2   cups sugar
4   cups boiling water
1   12-ounce can frozen
    pineapple juice concentrate
1   12-ounce can frozen
    lemonade concentrate
2   liters lemon-lime carbonated
    soft drink

Dissolve gelatin and sugar in boiling water. Stir in pineapple concentrate and lemonade concentrate, mixing until smooth. Pour into freezer-safe bowl and freeze overnight. Let stand at room temperature for 1 hour before serving. Add soft drink and scoop slush into individual glasses.

Serves 25.

STRAWBERRY SLUSH PUNCH

½   cup sugar
1   6-ounce can frozen orange
    juice concentrate
1   6-ounce can frozen lemonade
    or limeade concentrate
2   cups boiling water
1   10-ounce package frozen
    crushed strawberries
1   46-ounce can pineapple juice
1   liter ginger ale

Place sugar, orange juice concentrate and lemonade or limeade concentrate in large container. Add boiling water and stir until smooth. Add strawberries and pineapple juice. Divide punch between 2 1-gallon freezer bags and freeze. Let stand at room temperature until slushy. Pour ginger ale over slush and ladle into individual glasses.

Serves 30.

JUICE SPRITZER

4   cups cranberry-apple juice
1   cup orange juice
¼   cup lemon juice
1   28-ounce bottle carbonated
    water

Combine cranberry-apple juice, orange juice and lemon juice. Stir in water. Chill before serving.

Serves 8.

MINT TEA

Squeeze juice from lemons, reserving rinds. Combine lemon juice, sugar and cold water in pitcher. Combine lemon rinds, mint, tea and boiling water in saucepan. Bring to a boil, remove from heat and let stand for 6 minutes. Strain tea into pitcher of lemonade. Garnish individual servings with mint sprigs.

Serves 8.

4 lemons
1½ cups sugar
4 cups cold water
5 sprigs mint
5 tablespoons tea leaves, of choice
4 cups boiling water
   Mint sprigs

KENTUCKY FARM TEA

Combine lemonade concentrate, mint, tea bags and cold water in 2-quart pitcher, stirring with wooden spoon to bruise mint leaves. Steep for 24 hours in refrigerator. Remove tea bags and mint leaves. Stir and serve over ice.

Serves 8 to 12.

1 6-ounce can frozen lemonade concentrate, thawed, undiluted
1 cup packed mint leaves
4 tea bags
6 cups cold water

REFRESHING ICED TEA

Combine sugar, lemon juice and 2 cups boiling water. In separate container, combine tea, mint and remaining 2 cups boiling water. Steep both mixtures for 15 minutes. Remove mint and strain both mixtures. Add cold water.

Serves 8 to 12.

½ cup sugar
   Juice of 2 lemons
4 cups boiling water, divided
3 tablespoons Earl Grey tea leaves or 4 small tea bags
   Handful of mint leaves
4 cups cold water

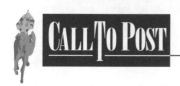

ICED TEA ELIXIR

2 cups sugar
2¼ cups water
Juice of 6 lemons
Juice of 2 oranges
Grated orange peel from
1 orange
1 cup packed mint leaves
Instant tea

Combine sugar and water in sauce-pan. Bring to a boil and cook until sugar is dissolved. Remove from heat and add lemon juice, orange juice, peel and mint. Cover and set aside until cool. Strain, then store in covered container in refrigerator. To serve, mix ⅓ cup elixir with ⅔ cup water and 1 to 2 teaspoons instant tea, mixing well.

Serves 12.

BOURBON SLUSH

1 cup sugar
2 cups hot tea
1 12-ounce can frozen
lemonade concentrate,
undiluted
1 6-ounce can frozen orange
juice concentrate, undiluted
6 cups water
1½ cups bourbon

Dissolve sugar in hot tea. Stir in lemonade and orange juice concentrates, water and bourbon. Pour into plastic container, cover and freeze for at least 24 hours. Serve as slush consistency.

Serves 16 to 24.

HOT RUM CIDER

If rum is used, reduce amount of cider to 7 cups.

8 cups cider
3 sticks cinnamon
Ground nutmeg to taste
Ground ginger to taste
1 cup rum (optional)

Combine cider, cinnamon, nutmeg and ginger in saucepan. Simmer for 5 minutes. Add rum and serve hot.

Serves 10 to 12.

MULLED CIDER

Using vegetable peeler, pare strips of peel from orange and lemon. Place peel, cinnamon, cloves and allspice on cheesecloth square, tie securely and place in large saucepan. Add cider, ginger ale, apples and brown sugar. Squeeze juice from orange and lemon and add to cider mixture. Bring nearly to a boil, reduce heat and simmer for 20 minutes, skimming foam from surface. Discard spice bundle. Pour 1 tablespoon brandy into individual mug, ladle cider into mug and garnish with ginger slices.

Serves 8.

½ orange
½ lemon
2 sticks cinnamon
5 whole cloves
3 whole allspice berries
5 cups apple cider
2 cups ginger ale
1 cup diced dried apples
½ cup firmly-packed brown sugar
1 cup Calvados brandy
8 crystallized slices ginger

PLANTER'S PUNCH

Combine lemon juice, lime juice, orange juice, pineapple juice, sugar, grenadine, soda, dark rum and light rum in large pitcher. Stir well. Pour punch into individual glasses each containing 4 ice cubes and garnish with orange slices and cherries.

Serves 4.

3 tablespoons fresh lemon juice
3 tablespoons fresh lime juice
¾ cup fresh orange juice
¾ cup pineapple juice
1 tablespoon superfine sugar
1 to 2 teaspoons grenadine
½ cup club soda
½ cup dark rum
½ cup light rum
4 orange slices for garnish
4 maraschino cherries for garnish

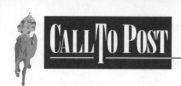

GRANDMOTHER'S EGGNOG

A delicious holiday treat! Beautiful served in a large punch bowl.

8   eggs, separated
½   cup bourbon
½   cup sugar
7   cups whipping cream
    Pinch of salt
    Ground cinnamon as garnish

Add bourbon to egg yolks, 1 tablespoon at a time, stirring gently to blend. Add sugar and mix; yolks will be light in color. Whip cream until peaks form. Separately whip egg whites with salt until peaks form. Fold whipped cream into egg yolk mixture, then fold egg whites into whipped cream, mixing until thick and smooth. Sprinkle individual servings with cinnamon.

Serves 30.

SALADS & DRESSINGS

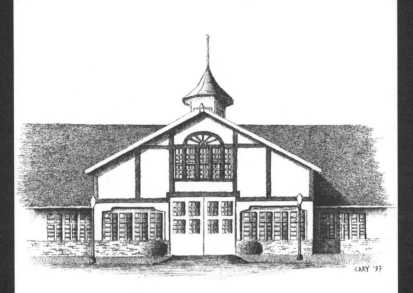

CARY '97

Since 1897, Xalapa Farm has been uniquely blessed with natural beauty and quite a history. Edward Francis Simms, son of noted Kentuckian William E. Simms, acquired these lands and created a place dedicated to the horse, while conserving the inherent beauty and preservation of the land. The Xalapa Training barn built in the early 1920's was designed by Edward F. Simms who drew plans for it in the dirt with his walking stick. This stone building has an eighth of a mile indoor track surrounding roomy stone and tile stalls. Large windows all around look out to the turn out paddocks. Down a scenic path is the one mile racetrack. Many champion horses started out here at Xalapa. For nearly a century, Xalapa has remained in the family as it is today.

Xalapa

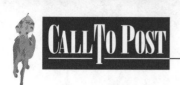

Salads & Dressings

Salad Dressings

Salads

Chicken

Fruit

Pasta

Seafood

Vegetable

NEW ORLEANS SEAFOOD SALAD

Combine vinegar, oil and mustard. Whisk until well blended.

DRESSING
⅓ cup red wine vinegar
⅔ cup vegetable oil
½ cup Creole mustard

Combine lettuce, tomatoes, crabmeat and shrimp. Prepare dressing, drizzle over salad and toss. Divide salad among 6 individual chilled plates. Press eggs through sieve. Garnish each salad with ½ sieved egg and 2 anchovies.

Serves 6.

SALAD
1 head iceberg lettuce, cored and torn in bite-sized pieces
2 large tomatoes, cored and cubed
1 pound backfin lump crabmeat
30 to 35 large shrimp, cooked, peeled and deveined
3 hard-cooked eggs
12 anchovies

FARFALLE PASTA SALAD WITH BRIE AND TOMATOES

A wonderful buffet salad.

Combine tomatoes, cheese, basil, garlic, oil, salt and black pepper. Let stand, covered, at room temperature for up to 4 hours. Prepare pasta according to package directions, cooking until tender but firm. Drain well. Add to tomato and cheese mixture, tossing to coat evenly. Serve at room temperature.

Serves 12 to 16.

4 ripe large tomatoes, seeded and diced
1 16-ounce round of Brie cheese, rind discarded and cut in 1-inch cubes
1 cup chopped fresh basil
1 teaspoon minced garlic
⅔ cup extra virgin olive oil
1 teaspoon salt
½ teaspoon freshly ground black pepper
1 16-ounce package farfalle (bow tie) pasta

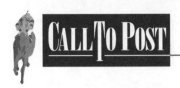
VEGETABLE AND CHICKEN PASTA WITH GRILLED TOMATO VINAIGRETTE

The perfect picnic dish.

SALAD
1   8-ounce package penne pasta
1   4-ounce boneless chicken breast
¼   cup plus 1 tablespoon minced green onion
¼   cup chopped red onion
1   medium red bell pepper, seeded and chopped
20 fresh snow peas, trimmed and cut in half
½   cup black olives, halved, or any oil-packed olives
1   14-ounce can artichoke hearts, drained and chopped

DRESSING
Dressing can be used on any green salad.
2   medium tomatoes, peeled, halved and seeded
2   teaspoons minced garlic
⅓   cup red wine vinegar
2   tablespoons lemon juice
1   teaspoon salt
1   teaspoon freshly ground black pepper
½   cup vegetable oil

Prepare pasta according to package directions, cooking until tender but firm. Rinse in cold water and drain well. While pasta is cooking, grill chicken and tomatoes (for dressing) over medium high heat; cook chicken until done and tomato halves until soft and slightly charred. Chill tomatoes until ready to use. Slice chicken. Combine chicken, pasta, green onion, red onion, bell pepper, snow peas, olives and artichoke hearts. Prepare dressing, drizzle half over salad and toss to coat evenly; add more dressing if preferred.

Combine grilled tomatoes, garlic, vinegar, lemon juice, salt and black pepper in food processor. Blend until smooth. With processor running, gradually add oil and blend until smooth.

Serves 6.

CHUTNEY CHICKEN SALAD

Blend mayonnaise and chutney together until smooth. Combine chicken, celery and green onion. Chop unpeeled apple, sprinkle with lemon juice and add to salad. Stir in grapes, pecans and brown rice. Fold mayonnaise mixture into salad, mixing lightly but thoroughly. Chill. Serve scoops of salad on lettuce.

Serves 6.

1   cup mayonnaise
½   cup chutney
8   boneless, skinless, chicken
    breast halves, cooked, cut in
    bite-sized pieces
2   stalks celery, chopped
4   green onions, chopped
1   Granny Smith apple
    Lemon juice
½   cup red seedless grapes
½   cup chopped pecans, toasted
2   cups cooked brown rice
    Lettuce leaves

CHILLED LENTIL SALAD

This is fabulous!

Cook lentils in boiling water for about 25 minutes or until tender. Drain well. Combine vinegar, shallots and mustard in large bowl. Gradually whisk in oil. Season with salt and black pepper. Add lentils and let stand until cool. Add cucumber, tomatoes, onion, dill, parsley and garlic. Season again with salt and black pepper. Chill, covered, for 1 hour. Crumble cheese over salad and mix lightly. Serve slightly chilled.

Serves 6.

SALAD
1   cup French green or brown
    lentils
    Water
2   tablespoons red wine vinegar
1   shallot, minced
1   tablespoon Dijon mustard
¼   cup olive oil
    Salt and black pepper to taste
1   cup diced cucumber, peeled
    and seeded
1   cup plum tomatoes, seeded
⅓   cup minced red onion
2   tablespoons chopped fresh
    dill
2   tablespoons chopped fresh
    parsley
1   large clove garlic, minced
1   6-ounce package soft goat
    cheese, crumbled

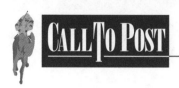

BROCCOLI SALAD

An easy year-around salad.

One small head cauliflower, broken in flowerets,
can be used instead of ½ portion of broccoli.

SALAD
2 **bunches broccoli flowerets,
    cut in bite-sized pieces**
1 **medium red onion, diced**
1 **cup shredded carrots**
½ **head purple cabbage,
    shredded**
1 **10-ounce package frozen
    baby peas, thawed**
1 **cup (4 ounces) shredded
    Cheddar cheese**
½ **cup raisins**
½ **pound bacon, cooked and
    crumbled**
1 **cup sunflower seeds**
¾ **cup chopped walnuts
    Lettuce leaves**

Combine broccoli, onion, carrots, cabbage, peas, cheese and raisins. Prepare dressing. Add to salad and mix well. Just before serving, add bacon, sunflower seeds and walnuts, tossing to mix. Pour salad into lettuce-lined bowl.

DRESSING
1 **cup mayonnaise**
½ **cup sugar**
3 **to 4 tablespoons cider or
    tarragon vinegar**

Combine mayonnaise, sugar and vinegar, whisking to blend.

Serves 6 to 8.

WARM BRIE DRESSING

2 **tablespoons walnut oil**
1 **tablespoon vegetable oil**
1 **8-ounce round of Brie cheese,
    rind discarded and cut in
    1-inch cubes**
2 **tablespoons sherry vinegar**
½ **cup whipping cream**
¼ **teaspoon salt**
¼ **teaspoon black pepper**

Combine walnut oil and vegetable oil in saucepan over low heat. Add cheese and cook, stirring to blend, until cheese is melted. Gradually whisk in vinegar, cream, salt and black pepper. Cook, stirring constantly, for about 10 minutes or until thoroughly heated.

Makes 1⅔ cups.

RED CABBAGE SALAD

A colorful summertime meal.

Cook potatoes in water in saucepan until tender. While potatoes are cooking, prepare cabbage. Using slicing blade in food processor, process cabbage until consistency for slaw. Prepare salad dressing, add to cabbage, toss to mix and place in large serving bowl. Layer ham, then cheese on cabbage. Drain potatoes and place on cheese. Sprinkle with pecans and drizzle with dressing. Serve immediately or later, at room temperature.

Combine mustard, cider vinegar, balsamic vinegar, honey, garlic, salt and black pepper in small bowl, whisking to blend. Gradually whisk in oil until it is emulsified. If not used immediately, store in covered jar in refrigerator. Shake vigorously before using.

Serves 8.

SALAD

1 **pound small new red potatoes**
1 **small head red cabbage, quartered**
1 **pound medium sliced honey baked ham, shredded**
1 **16-ounce package sliced Swiss Lorraine cheese, shredded**
½ **cup toasted pecans**

DRESSING

⅓ **cup grainy or stone-ground Dijon mustard**
¼ **cup cider vinegar**
¼ **cup balsamic vinegar**
3 **tablespoons honey**
¼ **teaspoon garlic**
    Salt and black pepper to taste
1 **cup virgin olive oil**

TOMATO SALAD WITH BALSAMIC VINAIGRETTE

A simple classic.

Arrange Bibb lettuce on individual plates. Place tomatoes on lettuce. Sprinkle green onion and cheese on tomatoes. Prepare vinaigrette. Drizzle over vegetables and cheese. Let stand at room temperature for 1 hour.

Combine vinegar, oil, mustard, salt and black pepper, whisking to blend well.

Serves 8.

SALAD

1 **head Bibb lettuce**
4 **large tomatoes, sliced**
3 **green onions, chopped**
1 **8-ounce package feta cheese, crumbled**

VINAIGRETTE

¼ **cup balsamic vinegar**
½ **cup olive oil**
1 **tablespoon dried mustard**
1 **teaspoon salt**
1 **teaspoon black pepper**

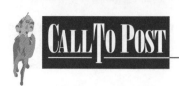

SUMMER POTATO SALAD

SALAD
6   medium potatoes, boiled and diced
5   tomatoes, cut in wedges
4   cucumbers, peeled and sliced
1   red onion, sliced
2   tablespoons chopped fresh dill
    Salt and black pepper to taste
    Lettuce leaves
    Sliced radishes for garnish

Combine potatoes, tomatoes, cucumber, onion and dill. Prepare dressing. Add to salad and mix well. Season with salt and black pepper. Chill, covered, for at least 3 hours. Serve salad on lettuce and garnish with radish slices.

DRESSING
    Juice of 2 lemons
½   cup sour cream
½   cup mayonnaise

Combine lemon juice, sour cream and mayonnaise, blending thoroughly.

Serves 8.

MARINATED TOMATOES

Perfect when tomatoes are at their peak.

6   tomatoes, peeled and sliced
2   tablespoons vegetable oil
¼   cup chicken broth
¼   cup red wine vinegar
1   tablespoon honey
¼   cup chopped parsley
¼   cup chopped green onion
1   clove garlic, minced
½   teaspoon salt
½   teaspoon freshly ground black pepper
½   teaspoon marjoram
½   teaspoon thyme
    Lettuce leaves

Place tomatoes in shallow dish. Combine oil, broth, vinegar, honey, parsley, green onion, garlic, salt, black pepper, marjoram and thyme. Pour dressing over tomatoes. Marinate, covered, for 24 hours. Drain tomatoes and serve on lettuce leaves.

Serves 8.

GRILLED VEGETABLE SALAD
WITH LEMON OREGANO VINAIGRETTE

Combine oil and red pepper flakes. Brush over eggplant, bell pepper, onion, zucchini and squash. Place vegetables on preheated grill and cook for 2 to 3 minutes on each side or until soft. Let stand until cool. Using vegetable peeler, shred ½ of Parmesan cheese; grate remaining cheese. Place endive on platter with grilled vegetables on top, sprinkle with chopped celery, carrot and radicchio. Drizzle with dressing. Prepare dressing. Sprinkle cheese shavings on salad.

SALAD
- ¼ cup olive oil
  Pinch of red pepper flakes
- 2 Japanese eggplant, cut lengthwise in halves
- 1 red bell pepper, cut lengthwise in ½-inch and seeded
- 1 small onion, cut in ¼-inch slices
- 1 zucchini, cut lengthwise in half ¼-inch slices
- 1 yellow squash, cut lengthwise in ¼-inch slices
- 1 4-ounce package Parmesan cheese
- 1 stalk celery, finely chopped
- 1 carrot, finely chopped
- 1 head radicchio, finely chopped
- 4 cups curly endive

Combine shallot, oregano, mustard and ½ of lemon juice, whisking to blend. Gradually add oil, whisking vigorously to mix. Add remaining lemon juice and season with salt and black pepper.

Serves 8.

DRESSING
- 1 shallot, peeled and minced
- 1 teaspoon fresh oregano, minced
- 1 teaspoon Dijon mustard
  Juice of 2 lemons
- ½ cup olive oil
  Salt and black pepper to taste

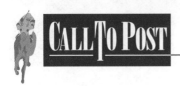

CALL TO POST

BREAD SALAD

Surprisingly delicious!

SALAD
- 3 pita bread rounds, split
- 4 lettuce leaves, shredded
- ½ cup chopped green onion
- 1 cup chopped cucumber
- 2 cups chopped tomatoes
- 1 bunch fresh mint leaves, chopped
- 1 bunch fresh parsley, chopped

DRESSING
Sumac can be found in specialty grocery stores.
- ½ cup lemon juice
- ⅔ cup olive oil
- 2 cloves garlic, minced
- 2½ teaspoons salt
- ½ teaspoon black pepper
- 1 tablespoon sumac

Split pita bread rounds and place on baking sheet. Bake at 350° until crisp. Break into 1-inch squares. Combine lettuce, onion, cucumber, tomatoes, mint and parsley in mixing bowl. Add pita squares and toss to mix. Prepare dressing, drizzle over vegetable mixture and toss. Correct seasoning, adding more lemon juice if necessary.

Combine lemon juice, oil, garlic, salt, black pepper and sumac, blending well.

Serves 6.

AUTUMN SPINACH SALAD

SALAD
- 1 bunch flat leaf spinach, coarsely chopped
- ⅓ cup currants or dried apricots
- 3 green onions, thinly sliced
- 1 green apple, cored and thinly sliced
- ½ cup seedless red grape halves
- ¼ cup chopped walnuts
- ⅓ cup crumbled goat cheese

DRESSING
- 2 tablespoons cider vinegar
- 2 tablespoons olive oil
  Salt and freshly ground black pepper to taste

Combine spinach, currants or apricots, green onions, apple, grapes and walnuts. Prepare dressing. Drizzle over vegetables and fruit, add cheese and toss to mix.

Combine vinegar and oil, blending well. Season with salt and black pepper.

Serves 3 or 4.

MIXED SALAD WITH POMMERY DRESSING

Combine spinach, raddichio, oranges, mushrooms and green onion. Prepare dressing. Drizzle over vegetables and toss to mix.

SALAD
1   bunch fresh spinach, torn in bite-sized pieces
1   head raddichio, torn in bite-sized pieces
3   oranges, peeled and sectioned
1   cup fresh mushrooms, sliced
½   cup chopped green onion

Combine vinegar, oil, chutney, garlic, mustard, sugar, salt and black pepper in tightly covered container. Shake well to blend.

Serves 6.

DRESSING
¼   cup wine vinegar
½   cup vegetable oil
¼   cup chutney
2   cloves garlic, minced
2   tablespoons pommery mustard
1   tablespoon sugar
    Salt and black pepper to taste

MIXED GREENS AND WALNUT SALAD

Toss walnuts with oil and season with salt and black pepper. Place on baking sheet. Bake at 350° for 4 to 6 minutes or until toasted; do not burn. Prepare dressing. Drizzle on greens and toss to mix. Place on individual chilled salad plates. Sprinkle walnuts and blue cheese on greens.

SALAD
1   dozen whole walnuts, broken in small pieces
1½   teaspoons walnut oil
     Salt and black pepper to taste
8   cups mixed greens
½   cup (2 ounces) crumbled blue cheese

Combine vinegar, shallot, olive oil, walnut oil, salt and black pepper, blending well.

Serves 4 to 6.

DRESSING
1   tablespoon red wine vinegar
1   small shallot, minced
3   tablespoons olive oil
2   teaspoons walnut oil
    Salt and black pepper to taste

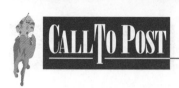

MIXED GREENS WITH WARM GOAT CHEESE SALAD

SALAD

- 2 heads Boston lettuce, torn in bite-sized pieces
- 2 heads Bibb lettuce, torn in bite-sized pieces
- 2 heads Romaine lettuce, torn in bite-sized pieces
- 3 bunches arugula, torn in bite-sized pieces
- 2 bunches watercress, torn in bite-sized pieces
- 1 bunch seedless grapes, cut in halves
- 1 16-ounce package goat cheese
  Chicken broth or olive oil
- 1 cup ground pecans
- ½ cup chopped parsley

Combine Boston lettuce, Bibb lettuce, Romaine lettuce, arugula, watercress and grapes. Cut goat cheese into 1x¼-inch rounds. Dip in broth or olive oil, roll in pecans, then in parsley. Place on baking sheet. Bake at 325° until toasted. Prepare dressing. Drizzle over vegetables and toss to mix. Scatter cheese rounds on salad and sprinkle with remaining pecans.

DRESSING

- ⅓ cup red wine vinegar
- 3 tablespoons walnut oil
- 2 tablespoons safflower oil
- ⅔ cup chicken broth
  Juice of 1 lemon
- 1 tablespoon Dijon mustard
- 2 to 3 green onions
- ½ teaspoon minced garlic
- 1 tablespoon sugar
- ¼ teaspoon salt
- ¼ teaspoon freshly ground black pepper

Combine vinegar, walnut oil, safflower oil, broth, lemon juice, mustard, green onions, garlic, sugar, salt and black pepper in blender container. Blend thoroughly.

Serves 8.

PEAR SALAD WITH RASPBERRY DRESSING

Toss pecans with butter. Place on baking sheet. Bake at 350° for 10 minutes. Let stand until cool. Dip pear slices in mixture of lemon juice and water to prevent discoloration. Combine Bibb lettuce and escarole. Prepare dressing. Drizzle on greens and toss to mix. Arrange pear slices on greens and sprinkle with pecans.

Combine oil, vinegar, preserves, sugar and mustard, whisking until smooth.

Serves 6.

SALAD
1   cup chopped pecans
3   tablespoons butter, melted
2   pears, thinly sliced
    Juice of 1 lemon
½   cup water
1   head Bibb lettuce, torn in bite-sized pieces
1   head escarole, torn in bite-sized pieces

DRESSING
¾   cup olive oil
¼   cup raspberry vinegar
2   tablespoons red raspberry preserves
¼   cup sugar
2   tablespoons brown mustard

MINT, STRAWBERRY, CUCUMBER SALAD

A light, colorful salad.

Combine mint and powdered sugar in small bowl. Using wooden spoon, crush mint to release flavor. Whisk in vinegar and oil. Add cucumber and marinate for 2 hours. Just before serving, stem and slice strawberries. On serving plate, alternately arrange cucumber and strawberry slices, beginning at outer edge of plate and spiraling toward center. Spoon remaining marinade over salad and season with black pepper.

Serves 8.

¼   cup chopped mint
2   teaspoons powdered sugar
¼   cup raspberry vinegar
½   cup olive oil
1   cucumber, thinly sliced
1   pound strawberries
    Freshly ground black pepper

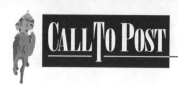

FRESH FRUIT SALAD WITH HONEY DRESSING

SALAD
- 2 medium peaches, peeled and sliced
- 1 cup diced fresh pineapple
- 1 cup honeydew chunks
- 1 cup blueberries
- 1 cup strawberries, sliced
- 2 medium bananas, diced
- 3 kiwi fruit, peeled and sliced

Combine peaches, pineapple, honeydew, blueberries, strawberries, bananas and kiwi. Prepare dressing. Drizzle over fruit and toss to mix.

DRESSING
- ⅔ cup sugar
- ¼ teaspoon salt
- 1 teaspoon dry mustard
- 1 teaspoon celery seed
- 1 teaspoon paprika
- 3 tablespoons vinegar
- 1 tablespoon lemon juice
- ½ teaspoon grated onion
- 1 cup vegetable oil
- ⅓ cup strained honey

Combine sugar, salt, mustard, celery seed and paprika. Blend in vinegar, lemon juice and onion. Gradually add oil, whisking to blend. Add honey and blend well.

Serves 8.

CREAMY GARLIC DRESSING

- 4 cloves garlic, minced
- 1 teaspoon salt
- 1 teaspoon freshly ground black pepper
- ½ teaspoon dry mustard
- 1 teaspoon Dijon mustard
- 1 egg
- 1 tablespoon fresh lemon juice
- ¼ cup balsamic vinegar
- ¼ cup extra virgin olive oil
- ½ cup vegetable oil

Combine garlic, salt, black pepper, dry mustard, Dijon mustard, egg, lemon juice, vinegar, olive oil and vegetable oil, blending thoroughly. Can be stored in refrigerator for up to 2 weeks.

Makes 1½ cups.

Soups

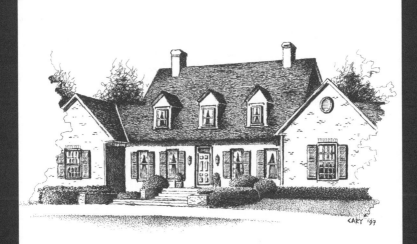

Since its inception in 1962, Mill Ridge Farm has grown from a small (four mares) Kentucky breeding operation to a full-scale commercial facility with extensive equine services. Sir Ivor, bred and sold by Mill Ridge in 1966, set the precedent for the next 30 years. Only the third American-bred winner of the Epsom Derby in 1968, Sir Ivor started a trend of American-bred classic winners in Europe, generating tremendous overseas interest in American yearlings.

Today, Mill Ridge is home to top stallions Gone West and Diesis, as well as Bien Bien, Binalong, Golden Gear and Valiant Nature. Located southwest of Lexington on Bowman Mill Road, Mill Ridge is within close proximity to Keeneland.

Mill Ridge

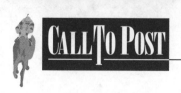

Soups

CHICKEN VEGETABLE SOUP WITH PESTO

Combine chicken, water, salt and black pepper in stock pot. Bring to a boil, reduce heat and simmer until chicken is tender. Drain chicken, reserving 8 cups broth. Remove skin and bones from chicken, cut into 1-inch pieces and set aside. Melt butter in stock pot over medium heat. Add onion, leek, carrot, celery, garlic, tomatoes, cabbage and green beans. Cook for 5 minutes. Stir in reserved broth, bring to a boil, reduce heat and simmer, uncovered, for 25 minutes. While soup is cooking, prepare basil pesto. Add spinach and chicken to soup. Simmer for 5 minutes. Remove soup from heat and blend in pesto. Serve in warm bowls and garnish each serving with Parmesan cheese.

Mash garlic with salt to form paste. Combine paste, basil, oil and cheese. Using food processor, blend until smooth.

Serves 4 to 6.

SOUP
4 chicken breast halves
9 cups water
  Salt and black pepper to taste
1 tablespoon butter
1 cup diced red onion
1 leek (white portion only), cleaned and cut in ¼-inch slices
1 carrot, cut in ½-inch slices
1 stalk celery, cut in ¼-inch slices
1 teaspoon minced garlic
4 Italian plum tomatoes, peeled, seeded and chopped
4 leaves cabbage, coarsely chopped
6 ounces fresh green beans, trimmed and cut in 1-inch lengths
10 large leaves spinach, torn in bite-size pieces
3 tablespoons basil pesto
  Freshly grated Parmesan cheese for garnish

BASIL PESTO
2 large cloves garlic
½ teaspoon salt
2 cups fresh basil leaves, washed and dried
⅔ cup olive oil
⅓ cup freshly grated Parmesan cheese

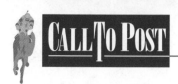

TORRES' CHILI BLANCO

2 cups dried Great Northern white beans
Water
6 chicken breast halves, skin removed
2 cups minced onion
2 tablespoons olive oil
4 cloves garlic, minced
6 Anaheim chilies, roasted, peeled, seeded and diced
1 jalapeño pepper, cored, seeded and minced
¼ teaspoon cayenne pepper
¼ teaspoon cloves
2 teaspoons ground cumin
1 tablespoon dried oregano
1 tablespoon fresh lime juice
Salt and black pepper to taste
2 cups (8 ounces) shredded Monterey Jack cheese
Chopped cilantro for garnish

Pour beans into large stock pot and add water to cover. Let stand for 1 hour. While beans are soaking, place chicken in large skillet and add 3½ cups water. Bring to a boil, reduce heat and simmer, covered, for 30 minutes. Drain chicken, reserving 3 cups broth. Remove skin and bones from cooled chicken, shred and set aside. Drain beans, discard liquid and set aside. Sauté onion in oil in stock pot over medium heat for 10 minutes. Add garlic, chilies, jalapeño pepper, cayenne pepper, cloves, cumin, oregano, reserved chicken broth, lime juice and beans. Bring to a boil, reduce heat and simmer, covered, for 2 hours. Season with salt and black pepper. Remove soup from heat. Add shredded chicken and cheese, stirring until cheese is melted. Garnish individual servings with cilantro. **Note:** Be sure to wear rubber gloves when handling jalapeño peppers.

Serves 8.

TORTILLA SOUP

Sauté onion, jalapeño pepper, garlic and turkey in stock pot until turkey is browned, stirring to crumble turkey and mix with vegetables. Add corn, tomatoes, tomato juice, broth, salt, black pepper, chili powder, cumin, Worcestershire sauce, hot pepper sauce and water. Bring to a boil, reduce heat and simmer, uncovered, for 1 hour. Stir in lime juice and tortilla strips. Simmer for additional 5 minutes. Sprinkle individual servings with cheese and garnish with chip mixture. **Note:** Be sure to wear gloves when handling jalapeño peppers. 2 to 3 cups chopped cooked chicken can be substituted for ground turkey.

Serves 8.

1	yellow onion, chopped
1	jalapeño pepper, chopped
2	cloves garlic, minced
1½	pounds ground turkey
2	cups frozen whole kernel corn
1	14½-ounce can chopped tomatoes or 2 fresh tomatoes, peeled, seeded and chopped
1	cup tomato juice
4	cups chicken broth
1	teaspoon salt
1	teaspoon black pepper
2	teaspoons chili powder
1	teaspoon ground cumin
2	teaspoons Worcestershire sauce
3	tablespoons hot pepper sauce
2	cups water
¼	cup fresh lime juice
4	corn tortillas, torn in strips
½	cup (2 ounces) grated Monterey Jack cheese Guacamole and/or salsa mixed with crumbled blue corn chips for garnish (optional)

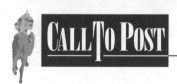

BUTTERMILK BROCCOLI SOUP

A hearty main course.

1   large onion, chopped
6   tablespoons butter, divided
4   cups fresh chicken broth
1   teaspoon salt
1   teaspoon freshly ground
     black pepper
1   teaspoon dried basil
1   bay leaf
1   teaspoon dried sage
1   teaspoon dried thyme
1   teaspoon hot pepper sauce
1½   pounds fresh broccoli,
     chopped
¼   cup plus 2 tablespoons all-
     purpose flour
1   cup milk
2   cups buttermilk

Sauté onion in 3 tablespoons butter in large saucepan until onion is softened. Stir in broth, salt, black pepper, basil, bay leaf, sage, thyme and hot pepper sauce. Bring to a boil, add broccoli, reduce heat and simmer, covered, for about 5 minutes or until broccoli is tender. In separate saucepan, melt remaining 3 tablespoons butter. Blend in flour and whisk until smooth and bubbly. Add milk and buttermilk. Stir until thickened. Combine sauce and broccoli broth, stirring until blended; do not boil.

Serves 6 to 8.

GAZPACHO

1   cucumber, peeled, seeded and
     chopped
½   green bell pepper, chopped
1   bunch green onions, chopped
2   very ripe tomatoes, seeded
     and chopped
1   very ripe avocado, peeled and
     cubed
4   cups tomato juice or Bloody
     Mary cocktail mix
3   tablespoons olive oil
2   tablespoons balsamic vinegar
½   teaspoon chopped fresh
     parsley
½   teaspoon dried oregano
     Salt and black pepper to taste

Combine cucumber, bell pepper, onion, tomatoes and avocado in large mixing bowl. Add tomato juice or Bloody Mary mix, oil, vinegar, parsley and oregano, mixing well. Chill, covered, for at least 4 hours before serving. Season with salt and black pepper.

Serves 4 to 6.

CREAM OF SPINACH SOUP

Delicious.

Wilt spinach by heating in skillet; do not add water. Place with natural liquid in food processor or blender and process for 10 seconds. Drain through sieve, reserving liquid, and set aside. Sauté onion in ¼ cup butter in large heavy saucepan over low heat until onion is transparent. Blend in flour, mixing until smooth. Add milk and whisk until smooth. Stir in spinach and liquid, salt, black pepper, nutmeg and cayenne pepper. Simmer for 3 minutes. In small bowl, beat egg yolks with cream. Very gradually add mixture to soup, stirring constantly to avoid curdling. Add parsley and 1 tablespoon butter and stir until butter is melted. Blend in lemon juice and serve immediately.

Serves 6 to 8.

2 pounds fresh spinach, washed and stems removed
2 tablespoons grated onion
¼ cup butter
3 tablespoons all-purpose flour
2½ cups whole milk, scalded
½ teaspoon salt
¼ teaspoon black pepper
¼ teaspoon nutmeg
Pinch of cayenne pepper
2 egg yolks
1 cup whipping cream
1 tablespoon minced fresh parsley
1 tablespoon butter
1 tablespoon fresh lemon juice

WILD RICE AND MUSHROOM SOUP

Sauté celery, mushrooms and onion in butter in large saucepan until celery is transparent. Reduce heat and blend in flour, stirring to form paste. Add broth and mix until smooth. Stir in chicken and wild rice. Cook until soup is thickened. Remove from heat and stir in half and half, sherry and lemon juice. Heat thoroughly but do not boil.

Serves 10.

1 cup chopped celery
1 cup sliced mushrooms
1 cup diced yellow onion
¼ cup butter
⅓ cup all-purpose flour
6 cups fresh chicken broth
1 pound cooked chicken, skin removed and cubed
2 cups cooked wild rice
1 cup half and half
3 tablespoons sherry
2 tablespoons fresh lemon juice

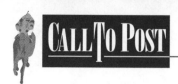

COLD TOMATO, BASIL AND WALNUT SOUP

Elegant!

3 pounds tomatoes, peeled and seeded
⅓ cup minced fresh basil
2 tablespoons walnut oil (no substitute)
1 tablespoon honey
2 tablespoons balsamic vinegar
2 teaspoons salt
1 teaspoon freshly ground black pepper
½ cup toasted chopped walnuts for garnish
Fresh basil sprigs for garnish

Purée tomatoes in food processor or blender. Combine tomatoes, basil, oil, honey, vinegar, salt and black pepper, mixing well. Chill thoroughly. Garnish individual servings with walnuts and basil sprigs. **Note:** Canned tomatoes can be substituted for fresh. Use 1 28-ounce can and 1 14½-ounce can; omit salt.

Serves 6.

WATERCRESS SOUP

1 yellow onion, chopped
1 bunch green onions, chopped
5 tablespoons butter
3 medium red skin potatoes, peeled and quartered
8 cups chicken broth
2 cups half and half
2 cups chopped watercress (without stems)
Salt and black pepper to taste
Watercress sprigs for garnish

Sauté yellow and green onions in butter in Dutch oven for 5 minutes. Add potatoes and broth. Bring to a boil, reduce heat and simmer until potatoes are tender. Add half and half and watercress. Simmer for 5 minutes. Remove from heat and purée mixture in food processor or blender. Season with salt and black pepper. Serve hot or chilled. Garnish individual servings with watercress sprigs.

Serves 6 to 8.

PIN OAK ASPARAGUS SOUP

A tradition.

Sauté onion in butter in large saucepan over medium heat until onion is transparent, stirring frequently. Add broth and bring to a boil. Trim tips from asparagus and reserve; trim 1 inch from opposite end of spears and discard. Cut remaining spear portion into 1-inch pieces and drop into boiling broth. Reduce heat and simmer, covered, for about 30 minutes. Remove from heat. Using about ⅓ at a time, purée in blender. Pour purée into saucepan, add reserved tips and simmer for about 5 minutes or until tender. Stir in half and half, hot pepper sauce, lemon juice, salt and black pepper. Heat for 5 minutes. Serve hot or chilled.

Serves 4.

2   cups chopped yellow onion
¼   cup unsalted butter
3½ cups chicken broth
1   pound fresh asparagus
½   cup half and half
1   tablespoon hot pepper sauce
2   tablespoons fresh lemon juice
    Salt and freshly ground black
    pepper to taste

CHILLED STRAWBERRY-RHUBARB SOUP

Combine strawberries, rhubarb and orange juice in saucepan. Simmer for 15 to 20 minutes. Remove from heat and stir in sugar and liqueur. Let stand until cool. Purée in blender with lime juice. Chill well. Serve cold, garnishing individual servings with mint leaves.

Serves 4 to 6.

2   cups fresh strawberries,
    stemmed
¾   pound fresh rhubarb, peeled
    and cubed
2   cups fresh orange juice
½   cup sugar
¼   cup orange liqueur
2   tablespoons fresh lime juice
    Fresh mint leaves for garnish

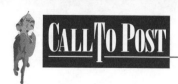

PEACH SOUP

½ cantaloupe, peeled and cubed
4 very ripe peaches, peeled and pitted
½ cup half and half
2 tablespoons Grand Marnier liqueur
2 tablespoons minced fresh mint leaves

Combine cantaloupe, peaches, half and half and liqueur in food processor or blender. Process until fairly smooth. Stir in mint. Chill well and serve cold.

Serves 4.

BLUEBERRY BISQUE

3 cups fresh blueberries
1 cup green seedless grapes
1 cup sour cream
4 teaspoons fresh lemon juice
1 teaspoon sugar
1 cup club soda
1 cup fresh orange juice

Purée blueberries and grapes together in food processor or blender. Strain through sieve into bowl. Whisk sour cream, lemon juice, sugar, club soda and orange juice into fruit mixture. Chill well and serve cold.

Serves 4.

CHEESE SOUP

1½ cups chopped cooked ham can be added to soup.

¾ cup finely chopped onions
½ cup finely chopped carrots
½ cup finely chopped celery
½ cup butter
½ cup all-purpose flour
2 tablespoons cornstarch
4 cups chicken broth
4 cups 1% milk
⅛ teaspoon baking powder
1 cup (5 ounces) firmly packed sharp Cheddar cheese
Salt and black pepper to taste
Fresh parsley sprigs for garnish

Sauté onion, carrots and celery in butter in large saucepan over low heat until softened. Blend in flour and cornstarch. Add broth and milk, mixing well. Cook, stirring often, until mixture is smooth and thickened. Add baking powder and cheese, stirring until cheese is well blended. Season with salt and black pepper. Garnish individual servings with parsley.

Serves 8.

CARROT SOUP

Easy to prepare.

Combine carrots, broth, butter, onions and potatoes in saucepan. Simmer for 25 minutes. Using slotted spoon, remove vegetables from liquid and place in food processor. Purée vegetables, then return to broth and reheat. Garnish individual servings with cheese.

Serves 4.

4   or 5 carrots, chopped
4   cups chicken broth
2   tablespoons butter
4   green onions, chopped
2   small potatoes, peeled and
    sliced
    Grated Gruyère cheese to
    garnish

SPLIT PEA SOUP

Soup freezes very well.

Combine broth, water, ham hocks and peas in large stock pot. Add onion, carrots, celery and garlic. Stir in peppercorns, cloves, thyme and bay leaf. Bring to a boil, reduce heat and simmer, partially covered, for 3 hours, stirring occasionally and skimming to remove froth. Remove and discard ham hocks and bay leaf. Process soup, in small batches, in food processor or blender. Return to clean stock pot. Stir in tomato paste, caraway seeds and lemon juice. Season with salt and black pepper. Soup should be very thick and hearty; thin with small amount of milk if necessary.

Serves 6 to 8.

4   cups chicken broth
4   cups water
2   or 3 ham hocks
1   16-ounce package green split
    peas, rinsed and sorted
1   medium onion, chopped
3   medium carrots, chopped
3   stalks celery, chopped
2   large cloves garlic, minced
4   peppercorns
3   whole cloves
½   teaspoon dried thyme
1   bay leaf
1   tablespoon tomato paste
2   teaspoons caraway seeds
1   teaspoon fresh lemon juice
    Salt and freshly ground black
    pepper to taste
    Milk (optional)

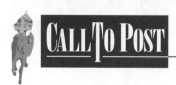

CREAMY ZUCCHINI SOUP

1 pound small zucchini, thinly sliced (unpeeled)
2 tablespoons finely chopped shallots or green onions
1 clove garlic, minced
2 tablespoons butter
¼ teaspoon curry powder
½ teaspoon salt
½ cup half and half
1¾ cups chicken broth

Simmer zucchini, shallots or green onions and garlic in butter in saucepan for 10 minutes, stirring occasionally. Pour mixture into blender and add curry powder, salt, half and half and broth. Blend for 30 seconds. Serve hot.

Serves 6.

LENTIL SOUP

2 medium carrots, sliced
2 medium stalks celery, sliced
1 medium onion, diced
1 clove garlic, minced
2 tablespoons olive oil
1 14½-ounce can Italian style stewed tomatoes
1 cup dry lentils
4 cups chicken broth
¾ pound red potatoes, diced
3 cups water
Salt and freshly ground black pepper to taste
½ pound fresh spinach, stemmed and thinly sliced

Sauté carrots, celery, onion and garlic in oil in 5-quart Dutch oven over medium heat for 5 to 8 minutes or until vegetables are tender. Stir in tomatoes, lentils, broth, potatoes and water. Stir with spoon to break up tomatoes. Season with salt and black pepper. Bring to a boil, reduce heat and simmer, covered, for 1 hour. Just before serving, stir spinach into soup and simmer for 10 minutes or until spinach is wilted.

Serves 6.

SWISS AND ONION SOUP

Sauté onion and garlic in butter in large saucepan until softened. Add mustard, salt and black pepper. Stir in broth. Simmer, covered, for 15 to 20 minutes. Combine milk and flour, whisking until smooth. Add to onion mixture, blending thoroughly. Stir in horseradish, sherry and cheese. After cheese is melted, add soy sauce, Worcestershire sauce and hot pepper sauce. Simmer for 5 to 10 minutes. Add kirsch and nutmeg just before serving.

Serves 4.

3   cups thinly sliced onions
1   clove garlic, minced
5   tablespoons butter
¾   teaspoon dry mustard
½   to 1 teaspoon salt
1½ teaspoons freshly ground black pepper
2   cups chicken broth
1½ cups milk
3   tablespoons all-purpose flour
½   teaspoon prepared horseradish
2   to 4 tablespoons dry sherry or more to taste
1½ cups (6 ounces) grated Swiss cheese
½   teaspoon soy sauce
½   teaspoon Worcestershire sauce
    Few drops hot pepper sauce
1   tablespoon kirsch
    Pinch of nutmeg

ORIENTAL CUCUMBER SOUP

Combine sherry, soy sauce and cornstarch, mixing thoroughly. Add to pork and stir to coat meat evenly. Sauté pork in oil in large Dutch oven over moderately high heat for 5 to 7 minutes, quickly browning meat. Add broth, reduce heat and simmer for 10 to 12 minutes. Stir in scallions, cucumber, salt and white pepper. Check seasoning. Simmer for 5 minutes, increase heat and bring to a fast boil.

Serves 6 to 8.

1   tablespoon dry sherry
2   tablespoons soy sauce
1   tablespoon cornstarch
½   pound lean pork, finely shredded
2   tablespoons vegetable oil
6   cups chicken broth
2   scallions with tops, sliced
1   medium cucumber, peeled, seeded and diced
1½ teaspoons salt
½   teaspoon white pepper

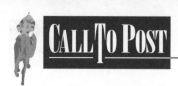

TWICE BAKED POTATO SOUP

10 slices bacon
1 cup diced yellow onion
½ cup finely chopped celery
½ cup chopped green onion
2 teaspoons minced garlic
1 cup all-purpose flour
6 cups hot chicken broth
5 cups baking potatoes, baked, peeled and diced
3 cups half and half
¼ cup chopped fresh parsley
2 teaspoons hot pepper sauce or to taste
2 cups (8 ounces) grated Cheddar cheese
1 8-ounce package cream cheese, cubed
3 tablespoons freshly grated Parmesan cheese
Salt and black pepper to taste
Grated Cheddar cheese for garnish
Chopped fresh parsley for garnish
Chopped scallions for garnish

Cook bacon in stock pot until crisp. Drain, crumble and set aside, reserving drippings in stock pot. Sauté yellow onion, celery, green onion and garlic in drippings over medium heat for 5 minutes. Add flour, blending until smooth. Gradually add broth and cook until thickened. Stir in potatoes and simmer for 15 minutes. Add half and half, parsley, hot pepper sauce, Cheddar cheese, cream cheese and Parmesan cheese. Cook, stirring constantly, until cheeses are melted. Season with salt and black pepper. Garnish individual servings with Cheddar cheese, parsley, scallions and bacon.

Serves 10.

BREADS

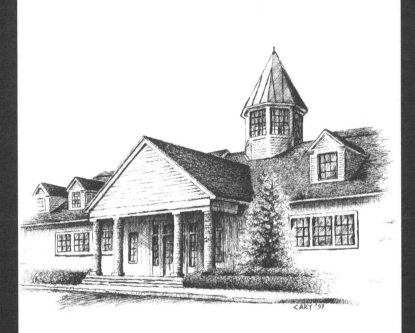

Owned by lifetime horseman William S. Farish and his wife Sarah, Lane's End is located on almost 2,000 acres in Woodford County in the heart of Central Kentucky. Internationally renowned for its stallion and sales divisions, Lane's End currently stands more than 20 stallions and has been the leading consignor for the past nine consecutive years at the prestigious Keeneland July sale. Lane's End and partners have bred and/or owned more than 190 stakes winners and such Champions as A.P. Indy and Storm Song were bred and sold by the farm. The farm also offers boarding, breaking, training, racing, and bloodstock services.

Lane's End

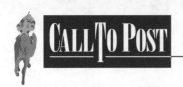

Breads

DELICIOUS APPLE BREAD

Combine apples, pecans and sugar, mixing well. Combine flour, soda, salt, allspice, cinnamon and nutmeg. Add dry ingredients and margarine to apple mixture. Combine eggs and vanilla. Add to apple mixture and mix well. Spread batter in 2 greased 9x5x3-inch loaf pans. Bake at 325° for 1 hour or until done. Cool in pan for 10 minutes, then remove to wire rack for cooling.

Makes 2 loaves.

4   cups diced peeled baking apples
1   cup finely chopped pecans
2   cups sugar
3   cups all-purpose flour
2   teaspoons baking soda
¼   teaspoon salt
¼   teaspoon allspice
1   teaspoon cinnamon
¼   teaspoon nutmeg
1   cup margarine, melted
2   eggs, lightly beaten
2   teaspoons vanilla

SOUR CREAM BANANA BREAD

Cream butter and sugar together until smooth. Add eggs and mix well. Sift flour, soda and salt together. Add dry ingredients, bananas, sour cream and vanilla to creamed mixture, blending well. Stir in pecans. Spread batter in greased 9x5x3-inch loaf pan. Bake at 350° for 1 hour. Cool in pan for 10 minutes, then remove to wire rack for cooling.

Makes 1 loaf.

½   cup butter, softened
1   cup sugar
2   eggs, beaten
1½ cups all-purpose flour
1   teaspoon baking soda
½   teaspoon salt
1   cup mashed bananas
½   cup sour cream
1   teaspoon vanilla
½   cup chopped pecans (optional)

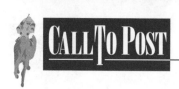

CRANBERRY CHEESE LOAF

2 3-ounce packages cream
   cheese, softened
2 eggs, divided
2 cups all-purpose flour
1 cup sugar
1½ teaspoons baking powder
¾ teaspoon salt
¾ cup apple juice
¼ cup butter, melted
1½ cups chopped cranberries
½ cup chopped nuts

Beat cream cheese until light and fluffy. Add 1 egg, blend well and set aside. Combine flour, sugar, baking powder and salt. Beat remaining egg and add with apple juice and butter to dry ingredients, mixing thoroughly. Fold in cranberries and nuts. Spread ½ of batter in greased and floured 9x5x3-inch loaf pan. Spoon cream cheese mixture evenly on batter and top with remaining batter. Bake at 350° for 65 to 75 minutes. Cool in pan for 15 minutes, then remove to wire rack for cooling. **Note:** Store in refrigerator or freezer.

Makes 1 loaf.

POPPYSEED BREAD

1 cup plus 2 tablespoons
   vegetable oil
1½ cups milk
3 eggs
1½ teaspoons almond flavoring
1½ teaspoons butter flavoring
1½ teaspoons vanilla
3 cups all-purpose flour
3 cups sugar
1½ teaspoons baking soda
1 teaspoon salt
2 tablespoons poppyseed

Combine oil, milk, eggs, almond flavoring, butter flavoring and vanilla. Combine flour, sugar, soda, salt and poppyseed. Using electric mixer, blend dry ingredients into egg mixture. Pour batter into 2 greased and floured 9x5x3-inch loaf pans. Bake at 350° for 50 to 60 minutes. Cool in pans for 10 minutes, then remove to wire rack for cooling.

Makes 2 loaves.

PUMPKIN BREAD

Sift flour, baking powder, soda, salt, cinnamon and nutmeg together in mixing bowl and set aside. Combine pumpkin, sugar, milk and eggs. Add to dry ingredients, stir in margarine or butter and mix well. Add pecans. Spread batter in 9x5x3-inch loaf pan. Bake at 350° for 45 to 55 minutes or until wooden pick inserted near center comes out clean. Cool in pan for 10 minutes, then remove to wire rack for cooling.

Makes 1 loaf.

2 cups pre-sifted, all-purpose flour
2 teaspoons baking powder
½ teaspoon baking soda
1 teaspoon salt
1 teaspoon cinnamon
½ teaspoon nutmeg
1 cup solid-pack canned pumpkin
1 cup sugar
½ cup milk
2 eggs, beaten
¼ cup margarine or butter, softened
1 cup chopped pecans

ZUCCHINI BREAD

Combine eggs, oil, sugar, zucchini and vanilla. In separate bowl, combine flour, baking powder, soda, salt and cinnamon, mixing well. Add dry ingredients to zucchini mixture and blend thoroughly. Stir in nuts. Spread batter in 2 greased 9x5x3-inch loaf pans. Bake at 325° for about 1 hour. Cool in pans for 10 minutes, then remove to wire rack for cooling.

Makes 2 loaves.

3 eggs, beaten until light and foamy
1 cup oil
2 cups sugar
2 cups grated zucchini
2 teaspoons vanilla
3 cups all-purpose flour
¼ teaspoon baking powder
1 teaspoon baking soda
¼ teaspoon salt
3 to 4 teaspoons cinnamon
½ cup chopped walnuts (optional)

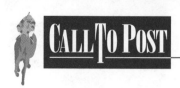

CALL TO POST

MRS. FANT'S COFFEE CAKE

½ cup vegetable shortening
1 cup sugar
¼ teaspoon salt
3 egg yolks
2 cups all-purpose flour
2 teaspoons baking powder
¾ cup milk
¼ teaspoon lemon extract
   Melted butter
   Powdered sugar, sifted
   Cinnamon

Cream shortening, sugar and salt together until smooth. Add egg yolks and blend well. Sift flour and baking powder together. Alternately add dry ingredients and milk to shortening mixture, beginning with dry ingredients. Stir in lemon extract. Spread batter in greased and floured 9-inch round baking pan. Bake at 350° for abut 40 minutes. Cool in pan for 5 minutes, then transfer to wire rack. Brush surface with melted butter and sprinkle with powdered sugar and cinnamon.

Serves 8.

OVERNIGHT COFFEE CAKE

2 cups all-purpose flour
1 cup sugar
1 cup firmly-packed brown
   sugar, divided
1 teaspoon baking powder
1 teaspoon baking soda
½ teaspoon salt
2 teaspoons cinnamon, divided
1 cup buttermilk
⅔ cup butter, melted
2 eggs
½ cup chopped pecans

Combine flour, sugar, ½ cup brown sugar, baking powder, soda, salt and 1 teaspoon cinnamon. Add buttermilk, butter and eggs. Using electric mixer, blend ingredients together at low speed, then beat at medium speed for 3 minutes. Spoon batter into greased and floured 13x9x2-inch baking pan. Combine remaining ½ cup brown sugar, 1 teaspoon cinnamon and pecans. Sprinkle on batter. Store, covered, in refrigerator overnight. Bake, uncovered, at 350° for 30 to 35 minutes.

Serves 12 to 16.

CINNAMON SWIRL BREAKFAST CAKE

For an extra treat, drizzle slices with honey and butter, then broil.

Sift flour, baking soda and salt together. Cream butter with 2¾ cups sugar until light and fluffy. Add eggs, 1 at a time, beating well after each addition. Stir in vanilla and lemon or almond extract. Using electric mixer, beat at high speed for 2½ minutes. Alternately add dry ingredients and buttermilk, beating at lower speed. Fold nuts into batter. Combine cinnamon and 2 tablespoons sugar. Spread ½ of batter in greased and floured 10-inch tube pan or 4 small loaf pans. Sprinkle ½ of cinnamon sugar on batter. Repeat layers. Using knife tip, swirl cinnamon mixture through batter. Bake at 325° for 1¼ hours.

Serves 16.

3	cups all-purpose flour
¼	teaspoon baking soda
¾	teaspoon salt
1	cup butter, softened
2¾	cups sugar
4	eggs
1	to 2 teaspoons vanilla
1	teaspoon lemon or almond extract
1	cup buttermilk
1	cup chopped nuts
2	tablespoons cinnamon
2	tablespoons sugar

CINNAMON STICKS

Cream butter and sugar together until smooth. Add egg yolk and beat well. Sift flour and cinnamon together. Add to creamed mixture and knead by hand until mixture holds together. Spread dough on ungreased 14x9-inch baking sheet and roll lightly with floured rolling pin to cover sheet. Lightly beat egg white and brush on dough. Sprinkle with nuts. Bake at 275° for 30 to 40 minutes or until lightly browned. Immediately after removing from oven, cut lengthwise into 3 strips, then cut crosswise into 1-inch pieces.

Makes 42.

½	cup butter, softened
1	cup sugar
1	egg, separated
1	cup all-purpose flour
2	teaspoons cinnamon
½	cup finely chopped nuts

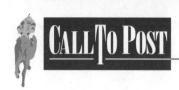

CREAM CHEESE BRAID

BREAD
- 1 cup sour cream
- ½ cup sugar
- 1 teaspoon salt
- ½ cup butter, melted
- 1 packet dry active yeast
- ½ cup lukewarm (105° to 115°) water
- 2 eggs, beaten
- 4 cups all-purpose flour

Heat sour cream in saucepan over low heat. Stir in sugar, salt and butter. Set aside to cool. In a medium size bowl, dissolve yeast in warm water. Add sour cream mixture, eggs and flour to yeast mixture, mixing well. Store, tightly covered, in refrigerator overnight. Prepare filling and glaze. Divide dough into 4 portions. Roll each on lightly-floured surface to form 12x8-inch rectangle. Spread ¼ of filling on each. Beginning at long edge, roll up in jelly roll fashion, pinch edges together, fold ends to enclose and place, seam side down, on greased baking sheet. At 2 inch intervals, cut slits ⅔ way through each roll. Cover and let rise until doubled in volume. Bake at 375° for 10 to 15 minutes. Spread glaze on rolls.

CREAM CHEESE FILLING
- 2 8-ounce packages cream cheese, softened
- ¾ cup sugar
- 1 egg, beaten
- ⅛ teaspoon salt
- 2 teaspoons vanilla

Combine cream cheese, sugar and egg. Stir in salt and vanilla.

GLAZE
- 2 cups sifted powdered sugar, sifted
- ¼ cup milk
- 2 teaspoons vanilla

Combine powdered sugar, milk and vanilla. Beat until smooth.

Serves 24.

FABULOUS FRENCH BREAD

So easy!

Combine yeast, sugar, salt and water in large bowl, mixing until dissolved. Stir in flour. Place dough in greased bowl, cover with damp towel and let rise in warm place for 45 minutes or until doubled in volume. Sprinkle cornmeal on greased baking sheet. Divide dough in 2 portions, shaping each into oblong loaf; do not knead. Place on baking sheet. Let rise 45 minutes or until almost doubled in volume. Brush tops of loaves with butter. Bake at 425° for 10 minutes, reduce oven temperature to 375° and bake for additional 20 minutes. Brush loaves with butter and serve hot.

Makes 2 loaves.

1 **packet dry active yeast**
1 **tablespoon sugar**
2 **teaspoons salt**
2 **cups lukewarm (105° to 115°) water**
4 **cups bread flour**
1 **tablespoon cornmeal**
  Melted butter

CRESCENT BUTTER ROLLS

Dissolve yeast with pinch of sugar in water; let stand until light and puffy. Combine butter, sugar, salt and milk. Blend in eggs. Add yeast liquid and mix well. Stir in flour, mixing to form sticky dough. Chill, covered, overnight. Divide dough into 3 balls and roll into 9-inch circles on lightly floured surface. Cut circles into 12 pie-shaped wedges and roll into crescent shapes. Place on baking sheet and let rise, uncovered, until doubled in volume. Bake at 375° for 12 to 14 minutes or until golden brown.

Makes 36.

1 **tablespoon dry active yeast**
  Pinch of sugar
¼ **cup lukewarm (105° to 115°) water**
¾ **cup butter, melted**
¼ **cup sugar**
1 **teaspoon salt**
1 **cup cold milk**
3 **eggs, lightly beaten**
4 **cups bread flour**

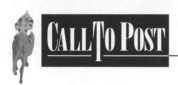

SPOON ROLLS

1 packet dry active yeast
1 teaspoon sugar
2 cups lukewarm (105° to 115°) water
¾ cup unsalted butter, melted
¼ cup sugar
1 egg, beaten
4 cups self-rising flour, unsifted

Dissolve yeast and 1 teaspoon sugar in water; let stand until bubbly. Blend butter with ¼ cup sugar. Add egg and beat well. Stir in yeast liquid and flour, mixing thoroughly. Place in airtight bowl and chill overnight. Drop batter by teaspoonfuls into greased miniature muffin pans. Bake at 350° for 15 minutes or until golden brown. **Note:** Batter can be stored in refrigerator for several days.

Makes 36.

YEAST ROLLS

1 packet dry active yeast
1 teaspoon sugar
¼ cup lukewarm (105° to 115°) water
⅔ cup sugar
1 teaspoon salt
½ cup vegetable shortening
1 egg, beaten
1 cup water
4 cups all-purpose flour

Dissolve yeast and 1 teaspoon sugar in water; let stand until bubbly. Using electric mixer, blend sugar, salt and shortening. Add egg, water and yeast liquid. Mix well. Blend in flour. Let rise, covered, until doubled in bulk. Punch down and shape dough into clover leaf or other shaped roll. Dip in butter, place in muffin pans and let rise until doubled in bulk. Bake at 400° for 10 minutes. **Note:** Dough can be stored in refrigerator for up to 7 days. For whole wheat rolls, use 2 cups white flour and 2 cups whole wheat flour.

Makes 36.

ANGEL BISCUITS

Dough can be stored in refrigerator for several weeks.

Dissolve yeast in water; let stand until bubbly. Sift flour, sugar, baking powder, soda and salt together. Using pastry blender or 2 table knives, cut shortening into dry ingredients. Stir in buttermilk and yeast liquid, mixing with spoon until all flour is moistened. Store, covered, in refrigerator until ready to use. Spread dough to ½-inch thickness, cut with biscuit cutter and place on baking sheet. Bake at 400° until browned.

Makes 40.

1	**packet dry active yeast**
½	**cup lukewarm (105° to 115°) water**
5	**cups all-purpose flour**
3	**tablespoons sugar**
1	**tablespoon baking powder**
1	**teaspoon baking soda**
1	**teaspoon salt**
¾	**cup vegetable shortening**
2	**cups buttermilk**

CHEESE 'N' DILL BISCUITS

Easy for a luncheon or tea.

Combine flour, baking powder, sugar, mustard and salt. Add butter and shortening. Using fingers, work mixture until it has consistency of coarse meal. Whisk milk, green onion and dill together. Add to dry mixture and stir until moist dough forms. Stir in 2 cups cheese. Place dough on lightly-floured surface and knead lightly to distribute cheese. Roll to ½ inch thickness. Using floured 2½-inch cookie cutter, cut biscuits and place on heavy ungreased baking sheet. Recombine scraps, roll and cut additional biscuits. Sprinkle cheese on biscuits. Bake at 450° for 15 minutes or until golden. Serve warm at room temperature.

Makes 18.

3	**cups all-purpose flour**
4½	**teaspoons baking powder**
1	**tablespoon sugar**
1½	**teaspoons dry mustard**
1	**teaspoon salt**
¼	**cup chilled unsalted butter, cut in pieces**
¼	**cup chilled vegetable shortening, cut in pieces**
1	**cup plus 2 tablespoons milk**
¼	**cup chopped fresh green onion**
3	**tablespoons packed chopped fresh dill or 1 tablespoon dried dill weed**
2½	**cups (10 ounces) grated extra-sharp Cheddar cheese, divided**

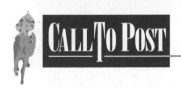

HONEY BRAN MUFFINS

2 cups all-bran
1 cup buttermilk
1 cup raisins
2 bananas
1 egg
¼ cup vegetable oil
¼ cup plus 2 tablespoons honey, divided
1 cup whole wheat flour
1 teaspoon baking soda
Pinch of salt
1 teaspoon cinnamon
¼ teaspoon nutmeg
2 tablespoons butter, melted

Combine bran, buttermilk and raisins. Let stand for 10 minutes. Mash bananas and add egg, oil and ¼ cup honey. Combine flour, baking soda, salt, cinnamon and nutmeg. Combine bran mixture, banana mixture and dry ingredients, mixing well. Spoon batter into greased muffin pan, filling cups ⅔ full. Bake at 375° for 18 to 20 minutes; do not overbake. Cool buns in pans for 5 minutes, then transfer to wire rack. Blend remaining 2 tablespoons honey with butter and drizzle over tops of buns.

Makes 12.

SOUTH OF THE BORDER CORN MUFFINS

1 cup all-purpose flour
1 cup yellow cornmeal
¼ cup sugar
1 tablespoon baking powder
1 teaspoon crushed red pepper flakes
1 egg
½ cup plus 1 tablespoon milk
¼ cup vegetable oil
1 17-ounce can cream style corn
2 or 3 jalapeño peppers, seeded and chopped

Combine flour, cornmeal, sugar, baking powder and red pepper flakes. Whisk egg, milk, oil and corn together. Pour liquids over dry ingredients and mix just until moistened. Spoon batter into generously greased muffin pans, filling 12 cups half full. Using back of teaspoon, make small depression in center of each muffin. Sprinkle small amount of jalapeño peppers in depression and top with remaining batter. Bake at 375° for 25 minutes or until light golden brown. Cool in pans for 2 minutes, then transfer to wire rack.

Makes 12.

CHEDDAR AND BACON MUFFINS

A hearty muffin and great served with a winter soup.

Cook bacon until crisp. Reserving 2 tablespoons bacon fat, drain slices, crumble and set aside. Cook scallions with salt, black pepper and caraway seeds in bacon fat over medium heat, until softened. Set aside to cool. Sift flour, baking powder, baking soda and sugar together. Whisk eggs, milk, mustard, shortening and scallion mixture together. Add dry ingredients and mix just until moistened. Stir in cheese and bacon. Spoon batter into greased muffin pans. Bake on center rack at 350° for 20 to 25 minutes or until wooden pick inserted near centers comes out clean. Remove muffins from pans and cool, right side up, on wire rack.

Makes 18.

1   pound bacon
1   cup finely chopped scallions
1   teaspoon freshly ground black pepper
1   teaspoon salt
1½ teaspoons caraway seeds
3   cups all-purpose flour
2   teaspoons baking powder
1   teaspoon baking soda
2   tablespoons sugar
2   eggs
1½ cups milk
3   tablespoons Dijon mustard
3   tablespoons vegetable shortening, melted and cooled
2   cups (8 ounces) coarsely grated extra-sharp Cheddar cheese

GOGO'S COCOA MUFFINS

For extra sweetness, dredge muffins in powdered sugar or cut cone from top of each, fill with sweetened whipped cream and replace cone.

Sift flour, sugar, cocoa and baking powder together. Using hands, blend butter or margarine into dry ingredients. Add milk and mix thoroughly. Spoon batter into greased muffin pans (8 large cups or 14 miniature cups). Bake at 375° for 20 minutes for large muffins and 15 minutes for miniature muffins.

Makes 8 or 14.

1   cup all-purpose flour
½   cup sugar
¼   cup cocoa
2   teaspoons baking powder
1   to 2 tablespoons butter or margarine
⅔   cup milk

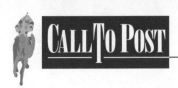

SWEET POTATO MUFFINS

1¼ cups mashed sweet potatoes
1¼ cups plus 2 tablespoons
    sugar, divided
½ cup butter, softened
2 eggs, at room temperature
1½ cups all-purpose flour
2 teaspoons baking powder
¼ teaspoon salt
1¼ teaspoons cinnamon, divided
¼ teaspoon nutmeg
1 cup milk
½ cup chopped raisins
¼ cup chopped pecans

Combine sweet potatoes, 1¼ cups sugar and butter. Beat until smooth. Add eggs, 1 at a time, beating well after each addition. Sift flour, baking powder, salt, 1 teaspoon cinnamon and nutmeg together. Alternately add dry ingredients and milk to sweet potato mixture, stirring just until moistened; do not overmix. Fold raisins and pecans into batter. Spoon batter into greased miniature muffin pans. Combine remaining 2 tablespoons sugar and ¼ teaspoon cinnamon. Sprinkle on batter. Bake at 400° for 25 to 30 minutes or until done. Serve warm. **Note:** Muffins can be frozen and reheated.

Makes 24.

COMPANY CORNBREAD

3 cups self-rising cornmeal
⅓ cup sugar
6 eggs
1½ cups vegetable oil
3 cups sour cream
2⅔ cups cream style corn
½ cup honey
1¼ cups butter, softened

Combine cornmeal and sugar. In order listed, add eggs, oil, sour cream and corn, beating well after each addition. Pour batter into greased 13x9x2-inch baking pan. Bake at 350° for about 30 minutes. For honey butter, blend honey with softened butter. Serve with warm cornbread.

Serves 12 to 16.

BREAKFAST & BRUNCH

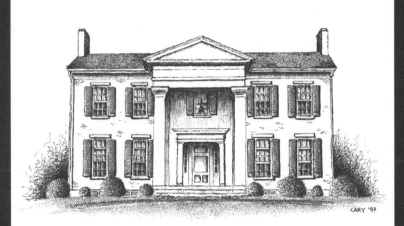

A family operation for over 50 years, Glencrest Farm comprises 1200 acres along the border of Scott and Woodford counties. Established by John W. Greathouse and now operated by his sons, John, Allen, David and Edward, they have bred over 75 stakes winners including Kentucky Derby winner Venetian Way, Kentucky Oaks winner Pike Place Dancer and champion Lady Pitt, all sold as yearlings by Glencrest at Keeneland. A full-service facility, Glencrest stands six stallions including Clever Trick and Wavering Monarch, and offers boarding and sales services.

Glencrest

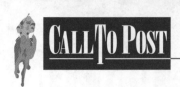

Breakfast & Brunch

DILLY SHRIMP AND EGGS

Melt butter in saucepan. Add green onion and water. Bring to a boil, reduce heat to medium and cook until water is evaporated. Stir in flour and cook for 3 minutes; do not brown. Add clam juice, wine, cream and dill. Cook, whisking constantly, until sauce boils. Blend in ½ cup Parmesan cheese. Remove from heat and set aside. Cut eggs lengthwise in halves. Place, yolk side up, in 13x9x2-inch baking dish. Spread shrimp on eggs. Pour sauce over shrimp. Combine bread crumbs, melted butter and remaining ½ cup Parmesan cheese. Sprinkle on sauce. Store in refrigerator until ready to bake, removing 30 minutes before baking. Bake, uncovered, at 400° for 20 minutes or until hot and bubbly. Garnish with dill sprigs.

Serves 8 to 10.

¼ cup butter
1 bunch green onions (1 inch green tops), thinly sliced
½ cup water
¼ cup plus 1 tablespoon all-purpose flour
½ cup clam juice
½ cup dry white wine
1 cup whipping cream
¼ cup minced dill or 2 teaspoons dill weed
1 cup (4 ounces) freshly grated Parmesan cheese, divided
16 hard-cooked eggs
1½ pounds shrimp, boiled with dill sprigs, peeled and deveined
1 cup dry bread crumbs
⅓ cup butter, melted
Dill sprigs (optional)

GLAZED CANADIAN BACON

Place bacon in baking dish. Press cloves in surface of bacon. Combine water and wine in saucepan and heat thoroughly. Pour over ham. Bake, covered, at 350° for 1½ hours. Blend jelly, vinegar, mustard and ground cloves to form sauce. During final 30 minutes of baking, brush sauce on bacon at 10 minute intervals. Slice thinly and serve warm with remaining sauce.

Serves 8.

1 32-ounce roll Canadian bacon Whole cloves
¾ cup water
¾ cup red wine
1 12-ounce jar currant jelly
1 tablespoon vinegar
1 teaspoon prepared mustard
½ teaspoon ground cloves

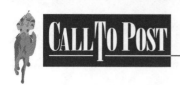

GREEN EGGS AND HAM

Assembled casserole can be stored, covered, in refrigerator
for up to 24 hours before baking.

2 tablespoons minced onion,
  divided
3 tablespoons butter
3 tablespoons all-purpose flour
½ teaspoon salt
2¼ cups milk, warmed
2 tablespoons dry sherry
3½ cups (14 ounces) shredded
  Cheddar cheese
3 10-ounce packages frozen
  chopped spinach, thawed
  and pressed dry
8 hard-cooked eggs
1 teaspoon Dijon mustard
3 tablespoons mayonnaise
1 teaspoon Worcestershire
  sauce
½ teaspoon salt
8 thin slices (6 inch rounds)
  baked ham

Sauté 1 tablespoon onion in butter in saucepan over medium heat until onion is translucent. Blend in flour and salt. Remove from heat and add milk, whisking to blend. Return pan to heat and, stirring constantly, bring to a boil and cook for 1 minute. Add sherry and Cheddar cheese. Cook over low heat, stirring occasionally, until cheese is melted. Mix 1½ cups cheese sauce with spinach. Spread spinach in 11x7x2-inch baking dish. Cut eggs lengthwise in halves, remove yolks and set whites aside. Mash yolks until smooth. Blend in remaining 1 tablespoon onion, mustard, mayonnaise, Worcestershire sauce and salt. Spoon yolk mixture into white halves. Place halves together to make whole eggs. Wrap ham slice around each egg, folding ends under. Place wrapped eggs on spinach, pressing slightly. Pour remaining cheese sauce over eggs. Bake, uncovered, at 350° for 35 to 45 minutes or until bubbly.

Serves 8.

GRAN'S EGG SIESTA CASSEROLE

Great served with Fruit Salad and muffins.

Assemble casserole the evening before. Place bread in buttered 13x9x2-inch baking dish. Spread chilies on bread. Combine eggs, milk, salt, garlic and oregano, mixing well. Pour egg mixture over chilies. Sprinkle Cheddar cheese and Monterey Jack cheese on egg layer. Store, covered, in refrigerator overnight. Bake at 325° for 50 minutes or until puffy and just firm. Serve immediately with avocado, cilantro, tomatoes or salsa and sour cream.

Serves 8 to 12.

8 slices bread
2 4-ounce cans chopped green chilies, drained
7 eggs, lightly beaten
2½ cups milk
1½ teaspoon salt
1 teaspoon minced garlic
1 teaspoon oregano
3 cups (12 ounces) grated sharp Cheddar cheese
3 cups (12 ounces) grated Monterey Jack cheese
½ cup sour cream
Avocado slices, for garnish
Chopped cilantro, for garnish
Chopped tomatoes or salsa, for garnish
Sour cream, for garnish

SIMPLY SENSATIONAL STRATA

Prepare broccoli according to package directions and drain well. Layer bread cubes, broccoli and ham in buttered 12x8x2-inch baking dish. Combine eggs, milk, onion, mustard and cheese, mixing well. Pour over layered ingredients. Chill, covered, for 24 hours. Bake, uncovered, at 325° for 55 to 60 minutes. Garnish with parsley, egg slices and paprika.

Serves 8.

1 10-ounce package frozen chopped broccoli
10 slices white bread, crusts trimmed and diced
2 cups diced cooked ham
6 eggs, lightly beaten
3½ cups milk
1 tablespoon minced onion flakes
¼ teaspoon dry mustard
3 cups (12 ounces) shredded sharp Cheddar cheese
Parsley sprigs for garnish
Hard-cooked egg slices for garnish
Paprika for garnish

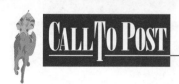

COUNTRY GRITS AND SAUSAGE CASSEROLE

2   pounds mild bulk pork
    sausage
4   cups water
1¼ cups uncooked quick-cooking
    grits
4   cups (16 ounces) shredded
    sharp Cheddar cheese
1   cup milk
½   teaspoon dried thyme
⅛   teaspoon garlic powder
4   eggs, lightly beaten
    Paprika
    Tomato wedges for garnish
    Parsley sprigs for garnish

Cook sausage in large skillet, stirring to crumble, until browned. Drain excess fat and set aside. Pour water into large saucepan and bring to a boil. Stir in grits, return to boil, reduce heat, cover and simmer for 5 minutes, stirring occasionally. Remove from heat. Add cheese, milk, thyme and garlic, stirring until cheese is melted. Add sausage and eggs. Spread mixture in lightly-greased 13x9x2-inch baking dish. Sprinkle with paprika. Bake at 350° for 1 hour or until golden brown. Let stand for 5 minutes before serving. Garnish with tomatoes and parsley. Note: Casserole can be assembled the evening before and stored, covered, in refrigerator overnight. Let stand at room temperature for 30 minutes before baking.

Serves 8 to 10.

GRANOLA

4   cups mixed oats, rye, barley,
    wheat and rice flakes
    Salt to taste
1   teaspoon nutmeg
½   cup honey
¼   cup butter, melted
1   cup coarsely chopped
    walnuts

Pour flakes into bowl and sprinkle with salt and nutmeg. Blend honey and butter. Pour honey syrup over flakes and toss until well coated. Spread mixture in single layer on aluminum-foil covered baking sheet. Bake at 300° for 20 to 30 minutes or until light golden, turning cereal every 10 minutes; do not overbake. Flakes will appear sticky but will dry when cool. Add walnuts after baking. Store granola in plastic bags or airtight container. Use within 1 month or store in freezer.

Makes 5 cups.

CHEESE SOUFFLÉ

Melt butter in heavy saucepan over low heat. Blend in flour and mix until smooth. Cook, stirring constantly, for 1 minute. Gradually add milk, salt, cayenne pepper, white pepper, mustard and Worcestershire sauce. Cook over medium heat, stirring constantly, until thickened and bubbly. Stir in Cheddar cheese. Remove from heat and let stand for about 10 minutes. Beat egg yolks until pale and thickened. Gradually stir ¼ of hot mixture into yolks, then add yolk mixture to remaining hot mixture, stirring constantly. Beat egg whites until stiff but not dry. Fold into cheese mixture. Spread in lightly buttered 2-quart soufflé dish. Place dish in 13x9x2-inch baking pan and add hot water to 1-inch depth in pan. Bake at 300° for 1½ hours. Serve immediately.

Serves 4 to 6.

3	tablespoons butter
¼	cup all-purpose flour
1¾	cups milk
1	teaspoon salt
¼	teaspoon cayenne pepper
¼	teaspoon ground white pepper
2	teaspoons prepared mustard
½	teaspoon Worcestershire sauce
1½	cups (6 ounces) sharp Cheddar cheese
6	eggs, separated

ORANGE MUFFINS

Cream butter and sugar together until smooth. Add egg and blend well. Dissolve soda in buttermilk. Add to egg mixture. Blend in flour and orange peel. Spoon batter into lightly-greased miniature muffin pan. Bake at 400° for 20 minutes. Combine orange juice and brown sugar. Spoon mixture over warm muffins, lifting each slightly to allow liquid to cover sides and bottom.

Makes 48.

1	cup butter, softened
1	cup sugar
2	eggs, lightly beaten
1	teaspoon baking soda
1	cup buttermilk
2	cups all-purpose flour
	Grated peel of 2 oranges
	Juice of 2 oranges
1	cup firmly-packed brown sugar

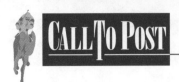
CHEDDAR GRITS PUDDING

Super!

4 cups water
1½ teaspoons salt
1 cup grits
½ cup yellow cornmeal
(preferably stone ground)
3 tablespoons unsalted butter,
cut in pieces
1 teaspoon sugar
¼ teaspoon cayenne pepper
2 teaspoons baking powder
½ cup milk
4 eggs, lightly beaten
1¼ cups (5 ounces) grated sharp
Cheddar cheese, divided
½ cup thinly sliced scallions
with green tops

Pour water into large heavy saucepan and bring to a boil. Stir in salt and gradually whisk in grits and cornmeal. Cook, covered, over low heat, stirring occasionally, for 25 minutes or until very thick. Remove from heat. Add butter, sugar and cayenne pepper. Stir until butter is melted. Dissolve baking powder in milk, add eggs and beat well. Add grits to egg mixture, mixing thoroughly. Stir in 1 cup of cheese and scallions. Spoon mixture into buttered 2-quart casserole. Bake at 325° for 1 hour. Sprinkle remaining ¼ cup cheese on pudding and bake for additional 15 to 20 minutes or until puffed and golden.

Serves 8.

CINNAMON BLINTZES

2 loaves thinly sliced fresh
white bread
2 8-ounce packages cream
cheese, softened
2 egg yolks
½ cup sugar
1 teaspoon lemon juice
1 cup firmly-packed brown
sugar
2 to 3 teaspoons cinnamon
1 cup margarine, melted

Trim crusts from bread. Roll slices to flatten. Combine cream cheese, egg yolks, sugar and lemon juice, mixing until smooth. Thinly spread cream cheese mixture on bread slices and roll up. Combine brown sugar and cinnamon in shallow bowl. Pour margarine into separate bowl. Dip rolls in margarine, then in brown sugar mixture and place close together on baking sheets. Freeze for 5 minutes. Slice each roll in half. Place rolls in plastic bags and freeze until ready to use. Place frozen rolls on greased baking sheet. Bake at 350° for 10 to 15 minutes.

Makes 64 to 80.

OATMEAL SOUFFLÉ

Combine milk and butter in small saucepan. Bring just to a boil. Gradually add oats, stirring constantly, and cook until thickened. Remove from heat and blend in cream cheese, brown sugar, salt, cinnamon and nutmeg, stirring briskly until smooth. Lightly beat egg yolks and gradually add to oatmeal, stirring constantly. Add raisins and walnuts. Beat egg whites until stiff but not dry. Using rubber spatula, gently fold egg whites into oatmeal; blend just until no large areas of whites remain and do not overmix. Spoon mixture into buttered and sugared 1½-quart soufflé dish or casserole. Bake at 325° for 35 to 40 minutes or until most of soufflé is set and center is slightly soft. Serve immediately with warm cream or milk.

Serves 4.

1	cup milk
2	tablespoons butter
¾	cup quick-cooking rolled oats
⅓	cup cream cheese
½	cup firmly-packed brown sugar
¼	teaspoon salt
½	teaspoon cinnamon
½	teaspoon nutmeg
3	eggs, separated
½	cup raisins
½	cup chopped walnuts
	Half and half or milk, warmed

BANANA PANCAKES

Combine flour and sugar. Blend in egg, milk and shortening. If batter is too thick, add small amount of milk. Fold bananas into batter. Ladle batter onto hot greased griddle or into skillet, placing 3 or 4 banana slices within each pancake. Cook, turn when bubbles appear and cook on second side until browned; cooking time may be slightly longer than regular pancakes. Sift or sprinkle powdered sugar on pancakes.

Serves 2.

1½	cups self-rising flour
3	tablespoons sugar
1	egg, beaten
¾	cup milk
3	tablespoons vegetable shortening, melted
1	large or 2 small bananas, sliced
	Powdered sugar, sifted

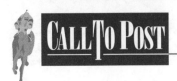

CLOUD PANCAKES

1 cup all-purpose flour
2 tablespoons sugar
2 tablespoons baking powder
½ teaspoon salt
1 egg
2 tablespoons vegetable oil
  Milk

Combine flour, sugar, baking powder and salt. Add egg, oil and enough milk to form pouring consistency. Mix lightly. Ladle batter on hot well-greased griddle. Cook, turn when bubbles appear and cook on second side until lightly browned.

Serves 2 or 3.

BEST SOUR CREAM PANCAKES

2 eggs, separated
2 tablespoons sugar
½ teaspoon baking soda
½ teaspoon salt
1 cup sour cream
1 cup sifted all-purpose flour

Beat egg yolks well. Add sugar, baking soda, salt and sour cream. Add flour and mix until smooth. Beat egg whites until stiff. Fold whites into batter. Drop batter by tablespoonfuls on hot ungreased griddle. Cook, turn when bubbles appear and cook on second side until lightly browned.

Serves 2 or 3.

OLD FASHIONED GRIDDLE CAKES

½ cup milk
2 tablespoons butter, melted
1 egg
1 cup all-purpose flour
2 tablespoons sugar
2 teaspoons baking powder
¼ teaspoon cinnamon

Combine milk, butter and egg, beating well. Mix flour, sugar, baking powder and cinnamon together. Add to liquid mixture and mix thoroughly. Ladle ¼ cup batter onto hot oiled griddle. Cook, turn when bubbles appear and cook on second side until browned. Serve on warm plate with maple syrup and sliced strawberries and blueberries.

Serves 2 or 3.

POPOVER PANCAKE

Heat well-greased 12-inch cast iron skillet in 425° oven for 5 minutes. Combine eggs, milk, flour, salt and melted butter or margarine, whisking to blend. Remove skillet from oven, pour batter into skillet and bake at 425° for 20 to 25 minutes. Pancake will resemble large popover but will fall quickly after removing from oven. Combine marmalade, 3 tablespoons butter or margarine and lemon juice in saucepan. Bring to a boil. Add peaches and cook over medium heat, stirring constantly, for 2 to 3 minutes. Spoon peach mixture on baked pancake and sprinkle with blueberries.

Serves 4.

4	eggs, lightly beaten
1	cup milk
1	cup all-purpose flour
¼	teaspoon salt
⅓	cup butter or margarine, melted
3	tablespoons orange marmalade
3	tablespoons butter or margarine
1	tablespoon lemon juice
1	16-ounce package frozen sliced peaches, thawed and drained
1	cup fresh or frozen blueberries

FANTASTIC FRENCH TOAST

Combine cream cheese and pineapple. Using electric mixer at medium speed, beat until light and fluffy. Stir in pecans. Cut bread into 12 slices, 1½ inches thick. Cut slit in crust in top of each slice and spoon cream cheese mixture into pocket. Combine eggs, cream, vanilla and ginger, whisking to blend. Dip bread slices in egg mixture, turning to coat on all sides. Cook slices on lightly-greased griddle over medium-high heat for 3 minutes on each side or until golden. Combine preserves and orange juice in saucepan. Warm over low heat, stirring constantly, until melted. Serve with hot toast.

Serves 6.

1	8-ounce package cream cheese, softened
¼	cup crushed pineapple
½	cup chopped pecans
1	16-ounce loaf French bread
4	eggs
1	cup whipping cream
½	teaspoon vanilla
1	teaspoon ground ginger
1	12-ounce jar apricot preserves
½	cup orange juice

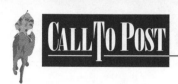

ORANGE MOUSSE

MOUSSE
2 packets unflavored gelatin
1½ cups sugar
⅛ teaspoon salt
4 egg yolks
2½ cups orange juice, divided
3 tablespoons lemon juice
1 tablespoon grated orange peel
2 11-ounce cans mandarin oranges, drained
2 cups whipping cream, whipped

FROSTED GRAPES
1 large bunch green or red seedless grapes
2 egg whites, lightly beaten
1 cup sugar

Combine gelatin, sugar and salt in saucepan. Beat egg yolks and 1 cup orange juice together. Stir into gelatin mixture. Cook, stirring constantly, over medium heat and bring to a boil. Remove from heat and stir in remaining 1½ cups orange juice, lemon juice and orange peel. Chill, stirring occasionally, until mixture mounds when dropped from spoon. Stir in oranges and fold in whipped cream. Pour into large ring mold. Chill until firm. Unmold on serving platter and garnish with frosted grapes.

Wash grapes and blot dry. Break into small clusters. Dip each cluster in egg whites, then place in plastic bag with sugar and toss to coat grapes. Place grapes on paper towel to dry. Arrange around mousse on platter.

Serves 12.

VEGETABLES

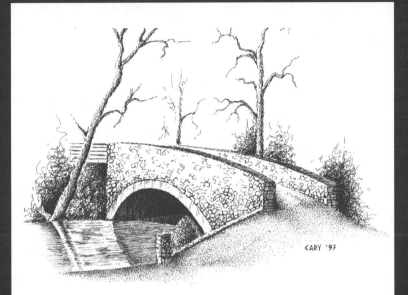

The walking bridges at Dixiana were built at the turn-of-the century as a passageway for horses to cross the historic Elkhorn Creek.

In 1877, the sign on the front gate read: "Nothing except a good race horse wanted. Agents for the sale of books, patent medicines, sewing machines, agricultural implements, horticulture and nursery products and *especially* of lightning rods and wire fences not admitted. Visitors of every nationality who will come unto my house always welcome."

— *B.G. Thomas*

Ownerships have changed, but the tradition continues: visitors are always welcome.

— *Pat & Bruce Kline*

Dixiana

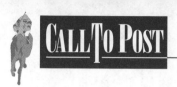

Vegetables

ARTICHOKE HEARTS WITH GRUYÈRE CHEESE

Prepare artichoke hearts according to package directions. While artichoke hearts are cooking, sauté garlic and shallots in butter and oil in large heavy skillet over low heat for about 5 minutes. Drain artichoke hearts and add with wine to garlic and shallots. Season with salt and black pepper. Cook over medium heat until wine is reduced to about 1 tablespoon. Remove from heat. Add Gruyère cheese and toss until cheese is melted. Garnish with parsley.

Serves 6.

2 9-ounce packages frozen artichoke hearts
2 cloves garlic, minced
¼ cup minced shallots
2 tablespoons butter
2 tablespoons olive oil
¼ cup dry white wine
   Salt and black pepper to taste
½ cup (2 ounces) grated Gruyère cheese
   Chopped fresh parsley for garnish

ASPARAGUS STIR FRY

Blanch asparagus in boiling water for 2 minutes, drain, plunge into ice water, drain and set aside. Heat oil in medium skillet over medium heat. Add mushrooms and sherry and cook for about 3 minutes. Stir in asparagus, snow peas, onion, soy sauce, oyster sauce and sugar. Season with salt and black pepper. Cook, stirring constantly, for about 3 minutes or until vegetables are tender and thoroughly heated. Blend cornstarch with cold water. Add to vegetables and cook until vegetables are glazed. Serve immediately.

Serves 4 to 6.

1 pound asparagus, peeled, trimmed and diagonally cut in 1-inch pieces
   Water
1 tablespoon vegetable oil
½ pound fresh mushrooms, stemmed and quartered
2 tablespoons dry sherry
6 ounces snow peas, trimmed
½ cup thinly sliced yellow onion
1 tablespoon soy sauce
1 tablespoon oyster sauce
1 tablespoon sugar
   Salt and freshly ground black pepper
1½ teaspoons cornstarch
1 tablespoon cold water

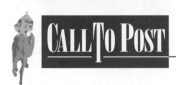

SESAME ASPARAGUS

So easy, a beautiful dish.

1½ pounds asparagus, peeled
and trimmed
Water
3 tablespoons butter
1 teaspoon sesame oil
1 tablespoon plus 1 teaspoon
fresh lemon juice
2 teaspoons soy sauce
3 tablespoons sesame seed,
toasted

Cook asparagus in boiling water in large skillet until tender. Drain, plunge into ice water, allow to cool, drain and blot dry. Melt butter and oil in skillet. Add lemon juice, soy sauce and sesame seed, mixing well. Drizzle mixture over asparagus and toss gently to mix.

Serves 6 to 8.

BAYOU RED BEANS AND RICE

1½ cups dried red beans, rinsed
and drained
Water
1 smoked ham hock
1 large onion, chopped
4 cloves garlic, minced
2 red bell peppers, chopped
and divided
3 tablespoons olive oil
6 tablespoons chopped parsley
3 cups chunky tomato sauce
2 teaspoons hot pepper sauce
Salt and black pepper to taste
4 cups cooked long grain white
rice
Parsley sprigs for garnish

Place beans in bowl, add water to cover and let stand for 4 hours. Drain beans, place in large saucepan with ham hock and add water to cover by 2 inches. Bring to a boil, reduce heat and simmer, uncovered, for 1 hour or until beans are tender. While beans are cooking, sauté onion, garlic and ½ of bell peppers in oil in large skillet over medium heat until vegetables are tender. Add vegetables, parsley, tomato sauce and hot pepper sauce to beans, liquid and ham hock. Simmer, uncovered, for 2 to 2½ hours or until thickened. Remove ham hock. Season with salt and black pepper. Spoon beans over individual servings of rice and garnish with remaining bell pepper and parsley.

Serves 6.

BAKED BEAN CASSEROLE

Great for cookouts or to take on a picnic.

Cook bacon and onion together in skillet until bacon is browned. Drain excess fat and set aside. Combine kidney beans, butter beans, pork and beans, ketchup, Worcestershire sauce and brown sugar. Stir in bacon and onion. Spread mixture in 9x9x2-inch baking dish and sprinkle with Cheddar cheese. Bake at 350° for 1 hour.

Serves 10 to 12.

6 slices bacon, diced
1 large onion, diced
1 16-ounce can red kidney beans, drained
1 16-ounce can butter beans, drained
2 16-ounce cans pork and beans, undrained
⅓ cup ketchup
¼ teaspoon Worcestershire sauce
½ cup firmly-packed light brown sugar
¼ cup (1 ounce) grated Cheddar cheese

WHITE BEANS WITH GARLIC

A great alternative to rice and potatoes.

Place beans in bowl, add water to cover generously and let stand overnight. Drain beans and place in large saucepan with 3 cups water and bay leaf. Bring to a boil, reduce heat and simmer, covered, for 1½ to 2 hours or until beans are tender, adding more water if necessary. Sauté garlic and onion in oil in heavy skillet over low heat for about 15 minutes or until translucent and golden. Add tomatoes, oregano and thyme. Simmer for 10 additional minutes. Drain cooked beans, add tomato mixture and season with salt and black pepper. Serve warm with extra olive oil.

Serves 6 to 8.

1 pound dried cannellini beans
Water
1 bay leaf
5 cloves garlic, minced
2 large onions, chopped
¼ cup olive oil
3 tomatoes, peeled, seeded and chopped
1 tablespoon chopped fresh oregano or 1½ teaspoons dried oregano
1 tablespoon chopped fresh thyme or 1½ teaspoons dried thyme
Salt and black pepper to taste
Olive oil

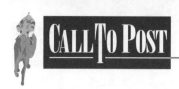

BLUEGRASS GREEN BEANS

1   pound green beans
    Water
⅓   cup coarsely chopped salted
    cashews or almonds
¼   cup butter
3   tablespoons honey

Cook green beans in boiling water until tender but crisp. Drain and cover to keep warm. Sauté cashews or almonds in butter in large skillet over low heat for about 5 minutes or until lightly browned. Add honey and cook, stirring constantly, for 1 minute. Pour sauce over beans and toss to coat thoroughly. Serve immediately.

Serves 3 or 4.

SPICED CAULIFLOWER

1   head cauliflower, cut in
    bite-sized pieces
    Water
1   clove garlic, chopped
2   tablespoons butter
2   tablespoons olive oil
    Salt to taste
    Ground nutmeg to taste
    Paprika to taste
    Chopped parsley for garnish

Steam cauliflower or cook in boiling water until tender. Drain and keep warm. Sauté garlic in butter and oil in large skillet for 2 minutes. Add cauliflower and sauté, turning to coat thoroughly. Cook, covered, for 3 to 5 minutes, shaking skillet occasionally. Season with salt, nutmeg and paprika. Sprinkle with parsley.

Serves 5 or 6.

BOURBON COUNTY CORN PUDDING

¼   cup all-purpose flour
3   cups fresh corn
2   tablespoons butter
2   eggs
½   teaspoon salt
½   teaspoon black pepper
1½   cups milk, cream or half and
     half

Combine flour and corn, mixing well. Combine butter, eggs, salt, black pepper and milk, cream or half and half in blender or mix by hand until frothy. Add to corn mixture, mixing thoroughly. Pour into greased 1½-quart casserole. Set casserole in pan of water. Bake at 300° for 1¼ to 1½ hours.

Serves 8.

BROCCOLI STIR FRY WITH LEMON-GARLIC SAUCE

Serve as side dish or with steamed rice for main course.

Cook broccoli in boiling water for about 2 minutes or until tender. Drain and set aside. Grate lemon peel to produce 1 teaspoon zest; halve lemon and squeeze to obtain 3 tablespoons juice. Combine zest, juice, soy sauce and sugar, mixing well. Blend in cornstarch until dissolved. Heat oil in wok or skillet until hot but not smoking. Add garlic, ginger and scallions. Stir fry for about 30 seconds or until garlic and ginger are fragrant. Add broccoli and lemon sauce. Stir fry for 1 to 2 minutes or until broccoli is thoroughly heated and sauce is thickened.

Serves 4.

5	**cups bite-sized broccoli flowerets**
	Water
1	**large lemon**
2	**tablespoons soy sauce**
2	**teaspoons sugar**
2	**teaspoons cornstarch**
2	**tablespoons vegetable oil**
2	**tablespoons minced garlic**
1	**teaspoon minced ginger root**
2	**tablespoons sliced scallions**

LENTILS WITH WALNUTS AND BACON

Combine lentils, bay leaf and ham hock in saucepan. Add water to cover. Bring lentils to a boil, reduce heat and simmer, uncovered, for 15 to 20 minutes or until lentils are tender. Drain, removing ham hock and bay leaf, set aside and cover to keep warm. Toss walnuts with 1 tablespoon walnut oil, salt and black pepper. Place on baking sheet. Bake at 350° for 5 to 8 minutes or until golden. Set aside. Whisk remaining 2 tablespoons walnut oil, vinegar, mustard, cayenne pepper and olive oil together. Combine warm lentils, walnuts, bacon, green onion and parsley. Drizzle with dressing, tossing gently to mix, and garnish with tomatoes.

Serves 6.

1½	**cups dried lentils, rinsed and drained**
1	**bay leaf**
1	**ham hock**
	Water
1	**cup chopped walnuts**
3	**tablespoons walnut oil, divided**
	Salt and black pepper to taste
¼	**cup red wine vinegar**
1	**tablespoon Dijon mustard**
⅛	**teaspoon cayenne pepper or to taste**
¼	**cup olive oil**
¼	**pound bacon, cooked, drained and crumbled**
½	**cup thinly sliced green onion**
3	**tablespoons chopped parsley**
4	**sun-dried tomatoes, thinly sliced (optional)**

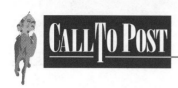

PEPPER JACK CORN BOATS

A different dish that you will make again and again.

4   ears unhusked sweet corn
1   cup chopped red onion
2   tablespoons olive oil
1   medium zucchini, cut ⅓-inch
    cubes
1   cup (4 ounces) coarsely grated
    Monterey Jack pepper cheese
2   tablespoons finely crushed
    corn tortilla chips

On each ear of corn, peel back a 1 to 1½-inch wide strip of husk to expose kernels and set strip aside. Peel back remaining husk, carefully keeping attached at stem end. Separate ear with kernels from husk at stem end, remove and discard silks and rinse. Using narrow strip from reserved husk, tie loose ends of each husk to form a boat shape and set aside. Cut kernels from ear and discard cob. Sauté onion in very hot (not smoking) oil in large skillet over moderate heat until lightly browned. Add zucchini and sauté until tender. Total cooking time for vegetables should be about 5 minutes. Remove from skillet with slotted spoon. Sauté corn in oil in skillet over medium heat for about 5 minutes or until tender crisp. Add to zucchini mixture and stir in cheese. Spoon into husk boats on baking sheet. Sprinkle with chips. Bake on upper rack at 375° for about 20 minutes.

Serves 4.

GLAZED CARROTS

2   cups sliced carrots
    Water
2   tablespoons butter
2   tablespoons orange
    marmalade
¼   teaspoon ground cinnamon
⅛   teaspoon ground nutmeg

Cook carrots in boiling water for 10 to 15 minutes or just until tender. Drain and keep warm. Combine butter, marmalade, cinnamon and nutmeg in saucepan. Add carrots and simmer for about 5 minutes or until well glazed.

Serves 3 or 4.

CORN ON THE COB WITH CHILI BUTTER

Peel husks back from corn without detaching from stem end. Remove silks and discard. Replace husks, smoothing around ear and tie ends together with string or strip of husks. Soak in cold water for 1 hour. Place chili powder in small saucepan or skillet, add butter and cook over medium heat, stirring, for 2 minutes. Add remaining butter and melt slowly. Remove from heat, skim any froth and set aside. Grill corn over medium-hot coals or heat for 15 to 20 minutes, turning often. If desired, peel back husks and cook corn directly on grill for a few additional minutes to brown kernels. Brush corn with chili butter and serve with lime wedges and salt.

Serves 6.

6 **ears yellow or white corn, unhusked**
1 **teaspoon chili powder**
½ **cup unsalted butter**
Lime wedges
Salt

QUICK AND EASY EGGPLANT PARMIGIANA

Serve with salad and crusty garlic bread for a simple supper or as a side dish for grilled chicken or pork.

Peel eggplant and cut into ¼-inch slices. Arrange slices in 1 layer, overlapping pieces, in 13x9x2-inch baking dish. Drizzle about 1 tablespoon olive oil over slices and sprinkle with cheese. Spoon spaghetti sauce over eggplant. Bake, covered with aluminum foil, at 350° for 45 minutes or until eggplant is tender.

Serves 4 to 6.

1 **medium eggplant**
Olive oil
2 **cups (8 ounces) grated mozzarella, asiago or other Italian cheese**
1 **32-ounce jar spaghetti sauce or 4 cups home prepared sauce**

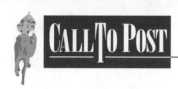

STUFFED ONIONS

Serve with beef tenderloin...a delight!

3 large onions
   Water
1 10-ounce package frozen
   chopped spinach, cooked and
   well drained
3 tablespoons mayonnaise
1 tablespoon lemon juice
½ cup (2 ounces) grated
   Parmesan cheese
   Salt and black pepper to taste

Parboil onions in water. Cut in halves, scoop pulp from centers, reserving shells, and chop pulp. Add spinach, mayonnaise, lemon juice and cheese to chopped onion. Season with salt and black pepper. Spoon mixture into onion shells and place in baking dish. Bake at 350° for 20 minutes.

Serves 6.

BISTRO ONION PIE

¼ cup butter, melted
1 cup finely crushed round
   buttery crackers
3 cups very thinly sliced onion
2 tablespoons butter
2 eggs, lightly beaten
⅔ cup milk
1 teaspoon salt
   Freshly ground black pepper
½ cup (2 ounces) shredded
   sharp Cheddar cheese

Pour melted butter into 9-inch pie plate. Add cracker crumbs and mix well with fork. Using spoon, press crumbs in bottom and along sides of pan to form crust. Set aside. Sauté onion in remaining 2 tablespoons butter in skillet over medium heat for about 12 minutes or until tender and translucent. Spread onions in crust. Combine eggs, milk, salt and black pepper in saucepan. Cook, stirring frequently, until hot; do not boil. Check and adjust seasonings. Pour sauce over onions and sprinkle with cheese. Bake at 350° for 30 minutes or until cheese is lightly browned. Cut in wedges and serve immediately.

Serves 4 to 6.

GRILLED VIDALIA ONIONS

Brush onion slices with ¼ cup vinaigrette and let stand for 15 minutes. Preheat barbecue grill to medium-hot. Brush slices with additional vinaigrette. Grill onion 4 inches from heat source for 3 to 4 minutes on each side, brushing with additional vinaigrette before and after turning. Slices should be brown and tender. Blend remaining vinaigrette with mustard, whisking until smooth and slightly thickened. Pour over grilled onions and serve immediately.

Serves 4 to 6.

2 large Vidalia onions, cut in 4-inch slices
¾ cup olive oil vinaigrette
2 tablespoons Dijon mustard

LEMON CAPER POTATOES

Potatoes are good accompaniment for beef or pork tenderloin.

Place potatoes in saucepan and cover with water. Bring to a boil and cook for 15 minutes or until tender. Drain, arrange slices on platter and keep warm. Sauté onion in butter in skillet over medium heat just until tender. Stir in lemon juice, caper juice, capers, parsley, salt and black pepper. Simmer until thoroughly heated. Pour sauce over potatoes, sprinkle with cheese and garnish with lemon slices.

Serves 8.

12 small new potatoes, unpeeled and sliced
    Water
2 tablespoons diced sweet onion
½ cup butter
¼ cup lemon juice
1 teaspoon caper juice
2 tablespoons chopped capers
2 tablespoons chopped parsley
1 teaspoon salt
¼ teaspoon black pepper
¼ cup (1 ounce) grated Parmesan cheese
    Lemon slices for garnish

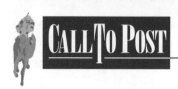

ROASTED PEPPERS

Peppers are especially good with drained anchovy fillets,
drizzled with olive oil and served with crusty Italian bread.

4   to 6 green or red bell peppers
2   or 3 cloves garlic, cut in
    halves
1   cup olive oil
    Salt and freshly ground black
    pepper
    Juice of ½ lemon

Char bell peppers over gas flame or under broiler until skins blister and blacken. Place in plastic container, seal tightly and let steam for 10 minutes. Peel skin from bell peppers, remove seeds and cut lengthwise into strips. Layer with garlic in bowl. Pour oil over vegetables. Season with salt, black pepper and lemon juice. Refrigerate, covered, for up to 1 week. Serve at room temperature.

Serves 6 to 8.

SWISS SCALLOPED POTATOES

Flavor is even better when dish is prepared in advance,
stored in refrigerator and reheated.

1½ cups (6 ounces) grated Swiss
    cheese, divided
½   cup chopped scallions
2   tablespoons unsalted butter
2   tablespoons all-purpose flour
1   teaspoon salt
1   cup 2% milk
1   cup low-fat sour cream
6   cups cooked cubed peeled
    potatoes
    Black pepper to taste
¼   cup fresh bread crumbs
¼   cup melted butter

Combine 1 cup Swiss cheese and scallions. Set aside. Melt 2 tablespoons butter in saucepan, blend in flour and salt and cook over low heat for 5 minutes to form roux. In separate pan, heat milk. Add to roux and cook, stirring often, to form béchamel sauce. Remove from heat and blend in sour cream. Spread 2 cups potatoes in buttered 3-quart casserole, season with black pepper, add ½ grated cheese mixture, then ½ sour cream mixture; repeat layers and top with remaining 2 cups potatoes. Combine remaining ½ cup Swiss cheese, bread crumbs and ¼ cup melted butter, mixing lightly. Sprinkle on potatoes. Bake, uncovered, at 350° for 40 minutes.

Serves 12.

BAKED POTATO SUPREME

This can be assembled in advance, stored in refrigerator and baked just before serving. It is a good accompaniment for beef tenderloin.

Cook potatoes in boiling water just until tender. Drain, let stand until cool and shred. Combine potatoes, sour cream and 1 cup Cheddar cheese. Add green onion, salt and black pepper. Spread mixture in buttered 2-quart casserole. Top with remaining 1 cup Cheddar cheese and sprinkle with paprika. Bake, uncovered, at 350° for about 35 minutes or until hot and bubbly.

Serves 10.

8 large potatoes, peeled and cut in bite-sized pieces
Water
2½ cups low-fat sour cream
2 cups (8 ounces) grated sharp Cheddar cheese, divided
1 bunch chopped green onion
2½ teaspoons salt
½ teaspoon black pepper
Paprika

SPINACH PIE

Place pastry in 9-inch pie plate, fold edges under and crimp along rim. Sauté onion in butter in large heavy skillet over medium heat for about 10 minutes or until tender. Blend in flour, spinach, salt, black pepper and nutmeg. Sauté until all liquid is evaporated. Combine ricotta cheese, mozzarella cheese and Parmesan cheese. Stir in eggs and add spinach mixture, blending well. Spoon mixture into pastry shell. Bake at 350° for about 45 minutes or until filling is firm at center and browned. Let stand for 10 minutes before cutting into wedges.

Serves 6.

1 unbaked 9-inch pastry shell, at room temperature
1 medium onion, chopped
3 tablespoons butter
1 teaspoon all-purpose flour
1 10-ounce package frozen chopped spinach, thawed and pressed dry
½ teaspoon salt
½ teaspoon black pepper
¼ teaspoon ground nutmeg
2 cups (15 ounces) ricotta cheese
1 cup (4 ounces) grated mozzarella cheese
1 cup (4 ounces) grated Parmesan cheese
3 eggs, lightly beaten

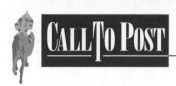

ORIENTAL SPINACH
Wonderful!!!

1 teaspoon minced garlic	Sauté garlic and ginger in oil and
1 teaspoon grated peeled	butter in large skillet over medium
ginger root	heat for about 30 seconds. Increase
1 tablespoon olive oil	heat to high, add spinach and cook,
1 tablespoon butter	stirring and turning to coat with oil
4 cups (about ¾ pound)	and butter, for about 1½ minutes or
spinach, stems removed and	until spinach begins to wilt. Sprinkle
washed	with soy sauce, sherry and sugar.
1 tablespoon soy sauce	Cook, stirring constantly, for about
1 tablespoon dry sherry	1 minute. Serve immediately.
1 teaspoon sugar	

Serves 4 to 6.

MEDITERRANEAN SPINACH PIE
Serve as a main course with salad and crusty bread.

2 bags spinach, stems removed, washed and blotted dry
2 medium onions, minced
½ teaspoon dill weed
6 eggs, well beaten
2 cups (8 ounces) crumbled feta cheese
1 cup small curd cottage cheese
¼ teaspoon white pepper
Dash of nutmeg
1 cup butter, melted, divided
10 sheets frozen phyllo dough, thawed

Combine spinach, onion, dill weed, eggs, feta cheese, cottage cheese, white pepper, nutmeg and ½ cup melted butter. Brush 14x10x2-inch baking pan with portion of remaining ½ cup melted butter. Brushing each sheet with additional butter, layer 4 sheets dough in pan. Spread ½ spinach mixture on phyllo. Again brushing each sheet with butter, layer 2 sheets dough on spinach. Spread remaining spinach mixture on phyllo. Top with 3 or 4 sheets dough, brushing each with butter. Trim edges and fold under. Using sharp knife, lightly score top dough layers. Bake at 350° for 1 hour.

Serves 6.

SPINACH SOUFFLÉ

Place spinach in greased 1-quart casserole and sprinkle with garlic powder, bacon and onion. Melt butter in saucepan. Blend in flour, salt and black pepper. Gradually add half and half and cook over medium heat until thickened, forming white sauce. Pour sauce over spinach and mix lightly. Bake at 350° for about 20 minutes or until bubbly.

Serves 4 or 5.

1	16-ounce package frozen chopped spinach, cooked and well drained
¼	teaspoon garlic powder
½	cup cooked chopped bacon
¼	cup minced onion
3	tablespoons butter
¼	cup all-purpose flour
½	teaspoon salt
½	teaspoon black pepper or to taste
1½	cups half and half

SOUTHERN SWEET POTATO RING

A great holiday dish.

Bake sweet potatoes at 350° for 1½ hours or until tender; potatoes can be cooked in microwave oven. Remove and discard skins, place in bowl and mash with fork. Add ½ cup butter, light brown sugar, milk, cinnamon, nutmeg, vanilla and egg, mixing well. Stir in raisins. Prepare 10-inch fluted tube pan or mold with vegetable cooking spray. Lightly grease with remaining 1 tablespoon butter. Sprinkle dark brown sugar in pan and add nuts. Spoon potato mixture into pan. Bake at 350° for 1 hour. Let stand for 15 minutes before inverting on warm serving dish.

Serves 12.

8	medium-sized sweet potatoes
½	cup plus 1 tablespoon butter, softened, divided
½	cup firmly-packed light brown sugar
1	5-ounce can evaporated milk
1	teaspoon cinnamon
1	teaspoon ground nutmeg
1	teaspoon vanilla
1	egg, lightly beaten
½	cup raisins (optional)
½	cup firmly-packed dark brown sugar
½	cup pecan halves

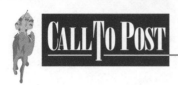

SWEET POTATO CASSEROLE

A departure from sweet potatoes with marshmallows!

3   cups mashed cooked sweet
    potatoes or yams
1   cup light corn syrup
¼   cup milk
⅓   cup butter, softened
2   eggs
1   teaspoon vanilla
1   cup coconut
1   cup chopped nuts
½   cup all-purpose flour
⅓   cup melted butter

Combine potatoes, syrup, milk, softened butter, eggs and vanilla, mixing well. Spread mixture in greased 9x9x2-inch baking dish. Combine coconut, nuts, flour and melted butter, mixing to form crumbs. Sprinkle evenly over potatoes. Bake at 350° for 30 minutes or until lightly browned.

Serves 6.

SPINACH STUFFED TOMATOES

Tomatoes can be prepared a day in advance, stored in refrigerator and reheated.

12   medium tomatoes
     Salt
2   10-ounce packages frozen
     chopped spinach
2   large onions, chopped
¼   cup chopped parsley
6   stalks celery, chopped
1   large green bell pepper,
     chopped
4   carrots, chopped
6   tablespoons butter
1½   cups seasoned bread crumbs
⅔   cup milk
2   eggs, beaten
     Salt and black pepper to taste
     Grated Parmesan cheese

Cut thin slice from tops of tomatoes. Scoop out seeds and pulp, setting aside for another use. Salt shells and invert to drain for 15 minutes. Prepare spinach according to package directions and drain well. Sauté onion, parsley, celery, bell pepper and carrots in butter in large skillet until onion is golden brown. Add drained spinach, bread crumbs, milk and eggs to sautéed vegetables. Season with salt and black pepper. Spoon mixture into tomato shells, packing firmly, and place in buttered baking dish. Sprinkle with Parmesan cheese. Bake at 400° for 20 minutes.

Serves 12.

FRESH TOMATO TART

Place pastry in 10-inch tart pan and prick with fork tines. Bake according to pastry package directions until done. Let stand until cool. Slice tomatoes and layer in crust, sprinkling with seasoned salt, black pepper and basil. Combine mayonnaise, Parmesan cheese, garlic and parsley. Spread mixture on tomatoes and sprinkle with crumbs. Bake at 400° for 15 minutes.

Serves 6 to 8.

1   unbaked 9-inch pastry shell
3   large ripe tomatoes
    Seasoned salt
    Freshly ground black pepper
1   tablespoon chopped fresh basil
½   cup mayonnaise
½   cup (2 ounces) grated Parmesan cheese
2   cloves garlic, crushed
½   cup chopped fresh parsley
¼   cup cracker crumbs

SPAGHETTI SQUASH ITALIANO

Bake squash at 350° for 1 hour or until tender when pierced with fork tines. Let stand for 5 to 10 minutes. Cut in half lengthwise and remove seeds. Using fork, pull spaghetti-like strands from shell and place in large serving bowl. Heat oil and butter in large skillet over medium heat. Add mushrooms, tomatoes, zucchini, green onion, garlic, bell pepper and snow peas. Cook for 4 to 5 minutes or until vegetables are softened. Pour sauce over squash strands and toss to combine. Sprinkle with Parmesan cheese and serve immediately.

Serves 4 to 6.

1   3 to 4 pound spaghetti squash
2   tablespoons olive oil
1   tablespoon butter
½   pound mushrooms, sliced
2   medium-ripe tomatoes, chopped
1   medium zucchini, cut in ¼-inch slices
5   or 6 green onions, chopped
1   teaspoon minced garlic
1   medium red bell pepper, cored, seeded and cut in ⅛-inch strips
¼   pound fresh snow peas, trimmed
¾   cup (3 ounces) freshly grated Parmesan cheese

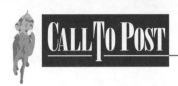

VEGETABLE BUNDLES

16　medium spears fresh
　　asparagus
2　carrots, cut in julienne strips
2　red bell peppers, cut in
　　julienne strips
8　green onions (green portion
　　only)
　　Salt and black pepper to taste
3　tablespoons butter, melted
4　teaspoons white wine

Trim asparagus to 2½-inch lengths, removing any woody portion or spots. Combine asparagus, carrots and bell pepper in steamer and steam until tender but firm. Trim any damaged tips from green onion tops and cut in 8-inch strips. Rinse and place in saucepan with water to cover. Cook for 1 minute over medium heat, drain and plunge into cold water. Assemble vegetable bundles, using 1 asparagus spear, 1 carrot strip and 1 bell pepper strip. Wrap each with onion strip and tie in bow at middle. Place bundles in buttered 3-quart casserole. Season with salt and black pepper. Drizzle with butter and wine. Bake at 350° for 10 minutes.

Serves 8.

BAKED SQUASH WITH ONION, BACON AND PARMESAN CHEESE

1　slice bacon, chopped
1　small onion, thinly sliced
2　pounds butternut or other
　　autumn squash, peeled,
　　seeded and thinly sliced
　　Salt and black pepper to taste
3　tablespoons freshly grated
　　Parmesan cheese

Combine bacon and onion in 13x9 x2-inch baking dish. Layer squash on onion and bacon and season with salt and black pepper. Bake, covered with aluminum foil, at 350° for 30 minutes or until squash is nearly tender. Remove foil, increase oven temperature to 400° and bake for additional 10 minutes. Sprinkle with Parmesan cheese and bake for about 10 additional minutes or until cheese is melted.

Serves 6 to 8.

SKILLET TOMATOES

Tomatoes, at peak of season, are a good accompaniment to steak.

Cut tomatoes in halves. Melt butter in skillet. Place tomatoes, cut surfaces down, in butter and sauté for a few minutes until golden brown. Blend vinegar, oil, salt, sugar, garlic and parsley. Turn tomatoes and add oil mixture. Simmer, tightly covered, for 15 to 20 minutes or until tender.

Serves 6 to 8.

- 4 large firm ripe tomatoes
- 1 teaspoon butter
- 1 tablespoon red wine vinegar
- 2 tablespoons olive oil
- 1 teaspoon salt
- 1 to 2 teaspoons sugar
- 1 clove garlic, pressed
- 1 tablespoon minced parsley

VEGETABLES VERSAILLES

Place onions on baking sheet. Alternately layer zucchini and yellow squash slices on onions. Place tomato wedges on squash. Drizzle with oil and season with garlic salt and black pepper. Bake at 325° for 45 minutes. Sprinkle with Parmesan cheese and broil until melted.

Serves 6 to 8.

- 3 large yellow onions, sliced
- 3 medium zucchini, thinly sliced
- 3 medium yellow summer squash, thinly sliced
- 3 or 4 tomatoes, sliced or cut in wedges
  Olive oil
  Garlic salt to taste
  Black pepper to taste
- ½ cup (2 ounces) grated Parmesan cheese

ZUCCHINI PUFF

Yellow squash or a combination of yellow and zucchini squash can be used.

Simmer zucchini in salted water for 5 minutes. Drain well. Combine zucchini, cottage cheese, Monterey Jack cheese, eggs and dill weed. Spoon mixture in shallow 1½-quart casserole. Bake, uncovered, at 350° for 15 minutes. Blend melted butter and bread crumbs, sprinkle on squash mixture and bake for additional 15 minutes.

Serves 6.

- 6 medium zucchini, cut in large pieces
  Water
  Salt
- 1 cup small curd cottage cheese
- 1 cup (4 ounces) shredded Monterey Jack cheese
- 2 eggs, beaten
- ¾ teaspoon dill weed
- 1 tablespoon butter, melted
- ½ cup fresh bread crumbs

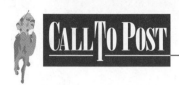

ZUCCHINI CASSEROLE

Great for a buffet dinner.

4 small zucchini, trimmed, shredded and blotted dry
1 medium onion, finely chopped
2 tablespoons olive oil
1 tablespoon cornstarch
2 eggs
1 cup half and half
¼ teaspoon hot pepper sauce
1 teaspoon salt
   Dash of freshly grated nutmeg
1 cup (4 ounces) shredded Gruyère cheese

Sauté zucchini and onion in oil in skillet for 5 minutes, stirring frequently. Sprinkle cornstarch over vegetables and cook for 1 minute. Remove from heat. Beat eggs, half and half, hot pepper sauce, salt and nutmeg together. Stir into zucchini mixture. Pour into greased 12x8x2-inch baking dish. Sprinkle with cheese. Bake at 400° for 25 to 30 minutes or until hot, bubbly and lightly browned.

Serves 8.

SUMMER SQUASH CASSEROLE

2 pounds yellow summer squash, sliced
½ cup sour cream
¼ cup butter, melted
¼ cup sliced green onion
½ teaspoon salt
⅛ teaspoon white pepper
1 cup cracker crumbs
¼ cup (1 ounce) freshly grated Parmesan cheese
¼ cup fresh minced basil
¼ cup fresh minced parsley
2 tablespoons fresh minced oregano

Steam squash until tender. Drain well. Combine squash, sour cream, butter, green onion, salt and white pepper. Spoon mixture into 1-quart casserole. Combine cracker crumbs, Parmesan cheese, basil, parsley and oregano. Sprinkle mixture on squash. Bake at 350° for 25 minutes.

Serves 6 to 8.

OKRA CORN TOMATO MEDLEY

Sauté onion in butter in Dutch oven until tender. Add okra and cook, stirring occasionally, for 5 minutes. Add corn, tomatoes, sugar, salt and black pepper, mixing well. Simmer, covered, for about 15 minutes or until corn is tender.

Serves 8 to 10.

1 medium onion, chopped
3 tablespoons butter
2 cups (about ½ pound) sliced okra
2 cups (about 3 medium ears) fresh corn kernels
3 cups (about 4 medium) tomatoes, peeled and chopped
1 teaspoon sugar
1 teaspoon salt
¼ teaspoon black pepper

STEAMED VEGETABLES WITH BASIL PECAN PESTO

Pesto can be stored in refrigerator for up to 1 week.

Mash garlic with salt to form paste. Combine paste, basil, oil, pecans and Parmesan cheese in food processor. Blend until smooth.

In steamer, place carrots on rack, add fennel and top with potatoes. Steam over boiling water for about 10 minutes or until potatoes are tender. Remove vegetables and keep warm. Steam green beans until tender. Add to other vegetables. Mix pesto with 3 tablespoons hot water, adding more to reach desired consistency. Serve warm or at room temperature with pesto.

Serves 6.

BASIL PECAN PESTO
2 large cloves garlic
½ teaspoon salt
2 cups fresh basil leaves, washed and blotted dry
⅔ cup olive oil
½ cup pecans, toasted brown and cooled
⅓ cup (1⅓ ounces) freshly grated Parmesan cheese

VEGETABLES
6 medium carrots, diagonally cut in ⅛-inch slices
2 bulbs fennel, stalks trimmed and bulb cut lengthwise in ⅛-inch slices
1½ pounds small red potatoes, cut in ¼-inch slices
Water
1½ pounds green beans, trimmed
3 tablespoons hot water

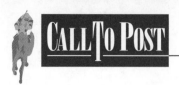

ROASTED RED PEPPER RATATOUILLE

Dish can be frozen. Use as side dish over couscous, rice or millet; on broiled or sautéed chicken breasts or broiled fish; in omelettes, on pasta or warmed on a roll and topped with melted goat cheese.

1 large eggplant, cubed
  Sea salt
3 red bell peppers
2 leeks, white portion only, chopped and well rinsed
2 medium onions, chopped
4 cloves garlic, minced
1 teaspoon sea salt
½ cup fresh minced basil
1 teaspoon oregano
2 tablespoons extra virgin olive oil
1 bay leaf
1 pound tomatoes, peeled
2 tablespoons tomato paste
1 cup tomato juice
2 tablespoons red wine
2 medium zucchini, cut in thin half-circles
3 tablespoons fresh chopped basil
1 tablespoon balsamic vinegar
  Salt and freshly ground black pepper to taste
2 tablespoons fresh chopped parsley

Toss eggplant with salt, place in colander and let drain for 1 hour. Rinse with cold water and press to remove all excess moisture. While eggplant is draining, roast or char bell peppers over gas flame or under broiler until skins blister and blacken. Place in plastic container, seal tightly and let steam for 10 minutes. Peel skin from bell peppers, remove seeds, cut lengthwise into strips and set aside. Sauté leeks, onion, garlic, 1 teaspoon sea salt, basil and oregano in oil in Dutch oven over medium heat for 5 to 10 minutes or until softened and translucent. Add bell pepper strips, eggplant and bay leaf. Simmer, stirring frequently, for 10 minutes. Add tomatoes, tomato paste, tomato juice and wine. Simmer for 15 minutes. Stir in zucchini and basil. Simmer for 15 to 20 minutes or until zucchini is tender but not soft. Add vinegar, mixing well, and season with salt and black pepper. Garnish with parsley.

Serves 6.

Pasta, Rice & Grains

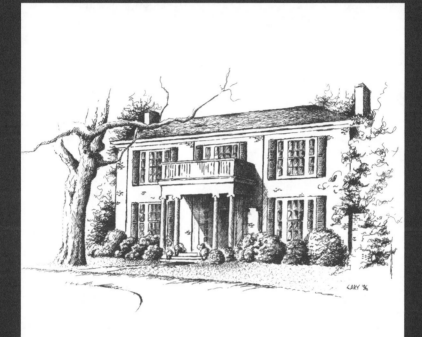

Established in 1974 by Mr. and Mrs. Robert Clay, Three Chimneys Farm is located in Woodford County ten miles northwest of Lexington on scenic Old Frankfort Pike. Three Chimneys is perennially one of the leading consignors at the prestigious Kenneland yearling sales and is home to champion stallions Seattle Slew, Arazi, Capote, Fly So Free, Slew o' Gold and world-class sires Wild Again, Rahy and Dynaformer, as well as promising newcomers French Deputy and Miesque's Son. On their one-thousand acre farm, the Clays board broodmares for clients from around the world.

Three Chimneys

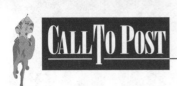

Pasta, Rice & Grains

FARFALLE WITH CHICKEN, BROCCOLI AND SUN-DRIED TOMATOES

Steam broccoli until crisp-tender and set aside. Drain tomatoes, blot dry with paper towel and cut into thin slices. Prepare pasta according to package directions, cooking until tender, yet firm. While pasta is cooking, sauté garlic in oil in skillet or saucepan until golden. Add chicken and sauté until cooked. Stir in broccoli and sauté for 1 minute. Add tomatoes, basil, red pepper, salt, black pepper, wine and broth. Blend in butter and simmer, covered, for 5 minutes. Remove from heat. Drain pasta, add to sauce and toss gently. Sprinkle individual servings with Parmesan cheese.

Serves 4.

2 cups broccoli flowerets
¾ cup oil-packed sun-dried tomatoes
1 8-ounce package farfalle (bow tie) pasta
3 cloves garlic, minced
¼ cup extra virgin olive oil
4 chicken breast halves, bone and skin removed and cut in ½-inch strips
¼ cup chopped basil or 2 teaspoons dried basil
Pinch of red pepper flakes
Salt and black pepper to taste
¼ cup dry white wine
¾ cup chicken broth
1 to 2 tablespoons butter (optional)
Grated Parmesan cheese

LEMON ASPARAGUS WITH FARFALLE

An ideal spring dish.

Prepare pasta according to package directions, cooking until tender but firm, and drain. Cook asparagus in small amount of water in saucepan for about 3 minutes or just until tender. Drain asparagus and mix with pasta. Add butter and toss to coat evenly. Keep warm in saucepan. Whisk egg yolks, cream and Parmesan cheese together. Add to pasta and asparagus. Simmer, stirring gently, until cheese is melted. Stir in chives, lemon peel, salt and black pepper.

Serves 4 to 6.

1 12-ounce package farfalle (bow tie) pasta
1 pound fresh asparagus, trimmed and cut in 1-inch pieces
2 tablespoons butter, melted
2 egg yolks
1¼ cups whipping cream
½ cup (2 ounces) grated Parmesan cheese
1½ tablespoons chives, chopped
2 teaspoons grated lemon peel
Salt and black pepper to taste

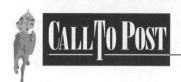

ORANGE AND FENNEL CHICKEN PENNE

A light, flavorful dish.

6   ounces boned, skinless chicken breast, cut in ½-inch cubes
2   tablespoons olive oil
1   large onion, chopped
3   cloves garlic, minced
1   10-ounce package penne pasta
1   small bulb fennel, cut in ½-inch chunks
½   cup orange juice
1   teaspoon orange zest
2   cups chopped tomatoes
½   cup chicken broth
3   tablespoons chopped fresh basil
¾   teaspoon salt
¼   teaspoon cayenne pepper
2   teaspoons cornstarch
1   tablespoon cold water
1   tablespoon pine nuts

Sauté chicken in oil in large skillet for 4 minutes. Transfer to plate and keep warm. Add onion and garlic to skillet and sauté for about 10 minutes or until translucent. Prepare pasta according to package directions, cooking just until tender. While pasta is cooking, add fennel to onion and garlic and stir in orange juice and zest. Cook, covered, for about 10 minutes or until fennel is tender. Stir in tomatoes, broth, basil, salt and cayenne pepper. Cook, uncovered, until slightly thickened, stirring frequently. Blend cornstarch and water to form smooth paste, add to sauce and cook until thickened. Add chicken and pine nuts. Drain pasta. Serve sauce over pasta.

Serves 4.

GRILLED CHICKEN AND PASTA WITH PESTO

Combine ¼ cup oil, lemon juice, minced garlic and black pepper in glass container. Place chicken in marinade and chill for several hours. Remove chicken from marinade and grill for 2 to 3 minutes on each side; do not overcook. Cut chicken in ¾-inch strips and keep warm. Prepare pasta according to package directions, cooking just until tender. While pasta is cooking, combine basil, ¼ cup Parmesan cheese, walnuts, 3 cloves garlic, parsley and white pepper in food processor. Process to pesto consistency. Drain pasta and return to cooking pot. Add pesto and chicken and mix gently but thoroughly. Sprinkle with Parmesan cheese.

Serves 4.

¾ cup extra virgin olive oil, divided
Juice of 1 lemon
2 cloves garlic, minced
Freshly ground black pepper to taste
4 chicken breast halves, skin and bone removed
1 12-ounce package corkscrew pasta
1 cup firmly-packed basil leaves, stems removed
¼ cup grated Parmesan cheese
2 tablespoons pine nuts
3 large cloves garlic
1 tablespoon parsley
¼ teaspoon white pepper
Grated Parmesan cheese

SPAGHETTI WITH SHRIMP SAUCE

This will quickly become a favorite.

Prepare pasta according to package directions, cooking just until tender but firm. While pasta is cooking, sauté onion in oil in large skillet over medium heat until translucent. Add shrimp and cook for 2 minutes, stirring constantly. Add wine and cook for about 2 minutes or until most of liquid is evaporated. Stir in tomatoes, season with salt and black pepper and cook for additional 2 minutes. Drain pasta and add to shrimp mixture. Blend in parsley and heat thoroughly. **For variety:** substitute cilantro for parsley.

Serves 6.

1 16-ounce package spaghetti
1 medium yellow onion, chopped
¼ cup olive oil
1¼ pounds large shrimp, peeled and deveined
⅓ cup dry white wine
1 14½-ounce can diced tomatoes, undrained
Salt and freshly ground black pepper to taste
¼ cup minced flat leaf parsley

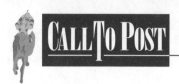

PENNE WITH GRILLED CHICKEN AND SPICY TOMATO SAUCE

½   cup olive oil, divided
     Juice of 1 lemon
7   cloves garlic, minced, divided
     Freshly ground black pepper
     to taste
6   chicken breast halves, skin
     and bone removed
½   teaspoon crushed red pepper
     or to taste
     Pinch of salt
1   14½-ounce can crushed
     tomatoes
1   14½-ounce can diced
     tomatoes, undrained
1   16-ounce package penne
     pasta
2   tablespoons vodka
1   cup whipping cream
¼   cup chopped parsley
     Freshly grated Parmesan
     cheese

Combine ¼ cup oil, lemon juice, 3 cloves garlic and black pepper in glass container. Place chicken in marinade and chill for 2 hours. Remove chicken from marinade and grill just until done. Cut into strips and keep warm. Combine remaining ¼ cup oil, 4 cloves garlic, red pepper and salt in large saucepan. Cook over medium heat for 2 to 3 minutes. Add crushed tomatoes and diced tomatoes. Simmer, uncovered, for about 15 minutes or until sauce begins to thicken. While sauce is cooking, prepare pasta according to package directions, cooking just until tender. Drain well and add to tomato sauce. Stir in vodka and cream. Add chicken and toss gently. Reduce heat and simmer, covered, for 1 to 2 minutes or until pasta partially absorbs sauce. Sprinkle with Parmesan cheese and parsley.

Serves 6.

LINGUINE WITH CHICKEN AND BROCCOLI

A great one-dish meal with tossed salad and bread.

Prepare pasta according to package directions, cooking until tender, yet firm. Drain and keep warm. Sauté chicken in olive oil in large skillet until no longer pink. Add onion and garlic. Sauté for 1 to 2 minutes. Stir in broccoli and ½ cup broth. Cook, covered, for 2 minutes; broccoli will be crisp. Combine remaining 1½ cups broth, lemon juice and cornstarch, blending until smooth, and add to chicken mixture. Add thyme, tomatoes and peas. Cook until sauce is thickened. Stir in almonds. Serve sauce over pasta. **Note:** Chicken breasts can be grilled, then cut into 1-inch cubes.

Serves 6.

1 **16-ounce package linguine**
6 **chicken breast halves, skin and bone removed, cut in 1-inch cubes**
3 **tablespoons olive oil**
¾ **cup chopped onion**
4 **cloves garlic, minced**
2 **cups chopped broccoli flowerets**
2 **cups chicken broth, divided**
1 **tablespoon lemon juice**
1 **tablespoon cornstarch**
2 **teaspoons fresh thyme or ¼ teaspoon dried thyme**
2 **14½-ounce cans diced tomatoes**
1½ **cups frozen peas**
¼ **cup sliced almonds, toasted (optional)**

FUSILLI WITH SAUSAGE, TOMATOES AND RICOTTA

Sauté onion in oil in large skillet over medium-high heat until softened. Add sausage and cook, crumbling with wooden spoon, until lightly browned. Stir in tomatoes and garlic. Season with salt and black pepper. Cook until tomatoes are reduced, about 10 minutes. Remove from heat and set aside. Prepare pasta according to package directions, cooking until tender but firm. While pasta is cooking, reheat sauce and stir in ricotta and basil. Drain pasta, pour sauce over pasta and toss, adding Parmesan cheese. Serve immediately.

Serves 4 to 6.

½ **cup minced yellow onion**
2 **tablespoons olive oil**
1½ **pounds mild Italian sausage, crumbled**
1 **14½-ounce can whole peeled tomatoes, undrained and coarsely chopped**
2 **cloves garlic, minced**
Salt and black pepper to taste
1 **16-ounce package fusilli pasta**
½ **cup whole-milk ricotta cheese**
¼ **cup torn fresh basil leaves**
¼ **cup (1 ounce) freshly grated Parmesan cheese**

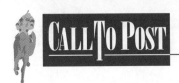

ANGEL HAIR PASTA WITH SHRIMP AND SCALLOPS

1   16-ounce package angel hair
     pasta
6   to 8 sun-dried tomato halves
½   cup white wine
1   medium onion, chopped
3   tablespoons olive oil
2   cloves garlic, minced
½   pound fresh shrimp, peeled
     and deveined
¼   pound sea scallops
1   10-ounce bunch spinach,
     washed and trimmed
3   tablespoons chopped fresh
     basil
¼   cup toasted pine nuts
     Salt and black pepper to taste
½   cup (2 ounces) grated
     Parmesan cheese

Prepare pasta according to package directions, cooking until tender but firm. Drain in colander and set aside. Combine tomatoes and wine in microwave-safe dish. Cook at high (100%) setting for 2 to 3 minutes or until tomatoes are rehydrated. Chop tomatoes and reserve liquid. Sauté onion in oil in large skillet until softened. Add garlic, shrimp and scallops. Sauté for 1 minute. Add spinach, cover and cook for 2 minutes. Stir in pasta, basil, pine nuts, salt and black pepper, tossing while cooking for 1 to 2 minutes or until thoroughly heated. Place in pasta serving bowls and sprinkle with remaining cheese.

Serves 6 to 8.

MOSTACCIOLI WITH MEAT SAUCE

2   cups chopped onion
½   cup chopped shallots
12   cloves garlic, minced
¼   cup olive oil
1   pound ground beef
1   pound ground veal
2   14½-ounce cans crushed
      tomatoes, undrained
1   14½-ounce can diced
      tomatoes, undrained
1½   cups chicken broth
1½   teaspoons dried oregano
½   teaspoon crushed red pepper
1   16-ounce package mostaccioli
      pasta
1   cup chopped fresh basil
      Freshly grated Parmesan
      cheese

Sauté onion, shallots and garlic in oil in large heavy saucepan over medium heat until vegetables are tender. Add beef and veal. Sauté over medium-high heat for 5 to 7 minutes or until cooked, stirring to crumble meat. Add crushed tomatoes, diced tomatoes, broth, oregano and red pepper. Bring to a boil, reduce heat and simmer for 20 to 25 minutes or until thickened. While sauce is cooking, prepare pasta according to package directions, cooking just until tender but firm. Drain pasta and place in pasta bowl or on large platter. Stir basil into sauce and pour sauce over pasta. Sprinkle individual servings with Parmesan cheese.

Serves 6 to 8.

PENNE WITH SHRIMP AND CHICKEN

Prepare pasta according to package directions, cooking just until tender but firm. While pasta is cooking, combine bread crumbs, ⅓ cup parsley, salt and black pepper in shallow bowl. Pour egg into separate bowl. Dip chicken in eggs, then in crumb mixture, turning to coat on all sides. Sauté chicken in 3 tablespoons oil in large heavy skillet for 4 minutes on each side or until cooked. Remove chicken and set aside; discard oil. Sauté shrimp with thyme in remaining 1 tablespoon oil over medium-high heat for about 3 minutes or just until cooked. Using slotted spoon, remove shrimp and set aside with chicken. Add wine to skillet, bring to a boil and cook for about 2 minutes or until liquid is reduced to ½ cup. Blend in cream and cook for about 3 minutes or until sauce is slightly thickened. Stir in red pepper and Parmesan cheese. Cut chicken into ½-inch pieces. Return chicken, shrimp and any collected juices to sauce in skillet. Stir over medium heat until heated thoroughly. Drain pasta, add to sauce and toss to coat thoroughly. Sprinkle with remaining 2 tablespoons parsley.

Serves 4.

1   8-ounce package penne pasta
2   cups fresh French bread crumbs
⅓   cup plus 2 tablespoons chopped parsley, divided
¾   teaspoon salt
½   teaspoon black pepper
2   eggs, beaten
¾   pound boned, skinless chicken breasts
¼   cup olive oil, divided
½   pound fresh large shrimp, peeled and deveined
1   tablespoon chopped fresh thyme or ½ teaspoon dried thyme
⅔   cup dry white wine
1   cup whipping cream
¼   to ½ teaspoon red pepper flakes
¼   cup (1 ounce) freshly grated Parmesan cheese

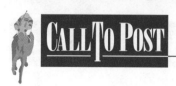

PIQUANT SEAFOOD SAUCE WITH PASTA

Citrus and spice combine for an interesting flavor.

1   carrot, diced
1   stalk celery, thinly sliced
3   large cloves garlic, minced
1   medium onion, chopped
3   tablespoons olive oil, divided
2   14½-ounce cans tomatoes,
    drained with ½ cup liquid
    reserved
1   teaspoon crushed red pepper
    flakes
1½ pounds medium shrimp,
    peeled, deveined and halved
    lengthwise
1   16-ounce package small shell
    pasta
¼   teaspoon saffron threads,
    crumbled
1   tablespoon hot water
½   teaspoon lemon zest
½   teaspoon orange zest
½   cup chopped basil leaves
    Salt and black pepper to taste
    Basil sprigs for garnish

Sauté carrot, celery, garlic and onion in 2 tablespoons oil in large saucepan until vegetables are softened. Drain tomatoes, reserving ½ cup liquid. Chop tomatoes in food processor, then add with reserved juice and red pepper flakes to sautéed vegetables. Simmer for about 10 minutes. While sauce is cooking, prepare pasta according to package directions, cooking just until tender. While pasta is cooking, sauté shrimp in remaining 1 tablespoon oil in medium skillet over high heat for 2 to 3 minutes or just until cooked. Set aside. Dissolve saffron in water and add with lemon zest, orange zest, basil, salt and black pepper to tomato sauce. Drain pasta and add to sauce, mixing thoroughly. Add shrimp and toss gently. Garnish with basil.

Serves 6.

LINGUINE AND SHRIMP WITH BASIL-MINT PESTO

The mint adds a refreshing twist.

Chop basil, mint, walnuts, Parmesan cheese and 1½ tablespoons garlic together in food processor. Gradually add 1 cup oil and process until smooth. Stir in red pepper flakes and set aside. Prepare pasta according to package directions, cooking just until tender but firm. While pasta is cooking, sauté shrimp with 1½ tablespoons garlic in remaining 2 tablespoons oil in large skillet over medium-high heat for 4 to 5 minutes or until shrimp is cooked. Drain pasta, reserving 1 to 2 tablespoons hot water, and place in bowl. Add shrimp. Blend reserved hot pasta water with pesto, spoon pesto over shrimp and pasta and toss well.

Serves 6 to 8.

4½	cups firmly-packed fresh basil leaves
1½	cups firmly-packed fresh mint leaves
¾	cup toasted walnuts, chopped
¼	cup plus 2 tablespoons (1½ ounces) grated Parmesan cheese
3	tablespoons minced garlic, divided
1	cup plus 2 tablespoons olive oil, divided
¼	teaspoon crushed red pepper flakes or to taste
1	16-ounce package linguine pasta
1½	pounds fresh large shrimp, peeled and deveined

MARINATED TOMATOES AND PASTA

A great no-cook sauce. Best when tomatoes are at their peak.

Combine fresh tomatoes, sun-dried tomatoes, garlic, oil, salt and black pepper. Let stand at room temperature for 1 hour. Prepare pasta according to package directions, cooking until tender but firm. Drain. Mix hot pasta with tomato mixture. Stir in basil. Serve warm or at room temperature.

Serves 4 to 6.

4	large ripe tomatoes, seeded and coarsely chopped
8	oil-packed sun-dried tomatoes, drained and coarsely chopped
3	cloves garlic, minced
½	cup olive oil
	Salt and freshly ground black pepper to taste
1	16-ounce package penne or linguine pasta
2	cups loosely-packed chopped fresh basil
	Grated Parmesan cheese (optional)

115

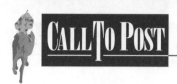

RIGATONI WITH SAUSAGE AND PEAS

A rich, hearty dish.

1 pound hot Italian sausage, casings removed
½ cup chopped onion
3 tablespoons olive oil
2 cups sliced fresh mushrooms
1 cup canned crushed tomatoes
1 14½-ounce can diced tomatoes, drained
1 tablespoon dried basil
1 teaspoon dried oregano
1 16-ounce package rigatoni
½ cup ricotta cheese, divided
1 cup half and half
1 cup fresh or frozen peas, thawed
   Salt and black pepper to taste
1 cup (4 ounces) grated Parmesan cheese

Fry sausage in heavy skillet, using back of wooden spoon to break into small pieces, until browned and thoroughly cooked. Remove sausage and drain on paper towels. Sauté onion oil in large saucepan or stock pot until translucent. Add mushrooms and cook for 3 minutes. Add crushed and diced tomatoes, basil and oregano. Simmer for 10 to 15 minutes or until sauce thickens slightly. While sauce is cooking, prepare pasta according to package directions, cooking until tender but firm. Add ¼ cup ricotta and half and half to sauce and boil gently for 3 to 4 minutes. Add sausage, peas and remaining ¼ cup ricotta. Season with salt and black pepper. Drain pasta and add with Parmesan cheese to sauce, mixing gently.

Serves 4 to 6.

SPAGHETTI WITH ROMANO CHEESE AND PEPPER

1 16-ounce package spaghetti pasta
¼ cup olive oil
2 cups (8 ounces) freshly grated Romano cheese
   Freshly ground black pepper (coarse grind)

Prepare pasta according to package directions, cooking until tender but firm. Drain and place in large bowl. Drizzle oil over pasta, add cheese and black pepper. Toss well and serve immediately.

Serves 4 to 6.

MANICOTTI FLORENTINE

Prepare pasta according to package directions, adding olive oil to boiling water. Cook until tender but firm. While pasta is cooking, wash spinach, blanch for 2 minutes, chop and squeeze to remove all excess moisture. Combine spinach, ½ of the mozzarella cheese, cottage cheese, feta cheese, egg, basil and pine nuts. Drain pasta shells. Pour 1½ cups tomato sauce into 13x9x2-inch baking dish. Spoon filling into pasta shells, place on sauce in dish, top with remaining 1½ cups sauce and sprinkle with remaining mozzarella cheese. Bake, loosely covered with aluminum foil, at 350° for about 50 minutes or until hot and bubbly.

Serves 4.

1	8-ounce package manicotti shells
1	tablespoon olive oil
1	bunch fresh spinach or 1 10-ounce package frozen chopped spinach, thawed
3	cups (12 ounces) grated mozzarella cheese, divided
1	cup small curd cottage cheese
1	cup (4 ounces) crumbled feta cheese
1	egg, lightly beaten
1	teaspoon dried basil
¼	cup toasted pine nuts, chopped
3	cups fresh or prepared tomato sauce

SPINACH FETTUCCINE WITH HOT PEPPER SAUCE

Prepare pasta according to package directions, cooking until tender but firm. While pasta is cooking, sauté garlic in oil in large skillet over medium heat until softened. Add tomato, basil, oregano and red pepper. Sauté for 5 minutes. Stir in bell pepper and sauté for about 5 minutes or until tender. Remove from heat. Stir in salt, black pepper, vinegar and olives. Drain pasta, add sauce and toss. Sprinkle Parmesan cheese on individual servings.

Serves 4 to 6.

1	16-ounce package spinach fettuccine
4	cloves garlic, minced
¼	cup olive oil
1	medium tomato, peeled, seeded and chopped
½	teaspoon dried basil
¾	teaspoon dried oregano
1	teaspoon dried crushed red pepper flakes
2	red bell peppers, cut in thin strips
	Salt and freshly ground black pepper
3	tablespoons red wine vinegar
¼	cup black olives, sliced
	Freshly grated Parmesan cheese

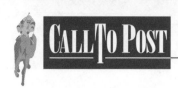

ELEGANT VEGETABLE LASAGNA

Worth the effort.

TOMATO HERB SAUCE

- ¼ cup butter
- ¼ cup all-purpose flour
- ¼ cup fresh minced basil
- ⅛ teaspoon dried oregano
- ⅛ teaspoon dried thyme
- 2 cups milk
- 1 10½-ounce can tomato puree
- 3 egg yolks
- ¼ teaspoon salt
- ¼ teaspoon freshly ground black pepper
- ¼ teaspoon cayenne pepper or to taste
- ¼ teaspoon ground nutmeg

Melt butter in saucepan over medium-low heat. When butter begins to bubble, whisk in flour, basil, oregano and thyme. Cook, stirring constantly, for about 5 minutes; do not allow flour to brown. Gradually whisk in milk, increasing heat to medium-high. Cook, stirring constantly, until sauce is thickened. Remove from heat and stir in tomato puree. Let cool for 5 minutes. Whisk in egg yolks. Add salt, black pepper, cayenne pepper and nutmeg. Pour into bowl and cover with plastic wrap.

LASAGNA

- 1 8-ounce package lasagna noodles
- 2 large onions, chopped
- ¼ cup butter
- 4 cloves garlic, minced
- ½ cup chopped almonds, toasted
- 5 10-ounce packages frozen spinach, thawed
- 2 4½-ounce jars sliced mushrooms, drained
- ¼ teaspoon salt
- ¼ teaspoon freshly ground black pepper
- ¼ teaspoon ground nutmeg
- 4 cups (16 ounces) regular or low-fat ricotta cheese
- ⅓ cup minced green onion
- 1 egg yolk, lightly beaten
- ¼ cup minced fresh basil
- ¼ cup minced fresh parsley

Prepare tomato herb sauce. Prepare pasta according to package directions, cooking until tender but firm. While pasta is cooking, sauté onion in butter in large skillet over low heat until very soft. Add garlic and almonds and cook for about 30 seconds. Press spinach to remove all excess moisture, add to onion mixture and cook until dry. Remove from heat and blend in mushrooms, salt, black pepper and nutmeg. Set aside. Combine ricotta cheese, green onion, egg yolk, basil and parsley, mixing well. In separate bowl, combine mozzarella, Parmesan and Swiss cheeses. Reserve 1½ cups of mixed cheese for topping. Drain pasta. Spread thin layer of tomato sauce in bottom of well-greased 13x9x2-inch baking dish. In order listed, layer ingredients: ¼ each of pasta, spinach mixture, ricotta cheese

(Continued on next page)

(Elegant Vegetable Lasagna, continued)

mixture and tomato sauce; repeat layers and top with reserved cheese mixture. Bake, loosely covered with aluminum foil, at 375° for 50 to 60 minutes or until hot and bubbly. Turn off oven and let lasagna stand in oven for 15 to 20 minutes. Cut into squares and serve.

Serves 8 to 10.

2½ cups (10 ounces) shredded mozzarella cheese
1½ cups (6 ounces) freshly grated Parmesan cheese
1 cup (4 ounces) shredded Swiss cheese

BASIC MARINARA SAUCE WITH PASTA

Delicious and so easy.

Sauté shallots in oil in large heavy saucepan over medium-low heat, stirring frequently, for about 3 minutes or until translucent. Add tomatoes and garlic. Cook, covered, stirring occasionally, for 20 minutes. Stir in basil and oregano. Simmer, uncovered, stirring frequently, for 15 to 20 minutes or until tomatoes are softened and liquid is evaporated. While sauce is cooking, prepare pasta according to package directions, cooking until tender but firm. Drain pasta. Season sauce with salt and black pepper. Just before serving, whisk in butter for richer flavor and smoother consistency. Serve sauce over pasta. Sprinkle individual servings with Parmesan cheese and parsley.

Serves 6.

3 tablespoons minced shallots
¼ cup olive oil
2 32-ounce cans Italian plum tomatoes, undrained and coarsely chopped
7 cloves garlic, minced
½ cup chopped fresh basil or 1½ tablespoons dried basil
1 tablespoon chopped fresh oregano or 1 teaspoon dried oregano
1 teaspoon marjoram (if using dried basil and dried oregano)
1 16-ounce package pasta
1 teaspoon salt
   Freshly ground black pepper to taste
2 to 3 tablespoons butter (optional)
⅓ cup (1⅓ ounces) freshly grated Parmesan cheese
   Chopped parsley

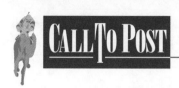
CORKSCREW PASTA WITH ROASTED ASPARAGUS AND LEMON

2 tablespoons pine nuts
2 pounds asparagus, trimmed and cut diagonally in 1-inch pieces
1 tablespoon olive oil
   Salt and freshly ground black pepper to taste
1 16-ounce package corkscrew pasta
1 cup chicken broth
2 tablespoons fresh lemon juice
1 tablespoon unsalted butter
¼ cup (1 ounce) freshly grated Parmesan cheese
2 tablespoons snipped chives
2 tablespoons chopped parsley
   Parmesan cheese for garnish

Place pine nuts in baking pan. Bake at 400° for 6 to 8 minutes or until golden. Remove nuts from pan and set aside. Increase oven temperature to 450°. Prepare pasta according to package directions, cooking until almost tender but very firm. While pasta is cooking, toss asparagus with oil and season with salt and black pepper. Place on baking sheet in single layer. Bake, tossing several times, for about 15 minutes or until browned; avoid burning. If asparagus is very thin, reduce baking time. Set aside. Drain pasta and combine with broth and lemon juice in large sauté pan. Cook over high heat for about 5 minutes or until liquid is nearly absorbed. Add butter, Parmesan cheese, asparagus, salt and black pepper. Cook, tossing or stirring, until butter is melted. Stir in chives and parsley. Using vegetable peeler, shave Parmesan cheese. Sprinkle cheese and pine nuts on individual servings.

Serves 4 to 6.

LINGUINE WITH SPINACH AND SUN-DRIED TOMATOES

A crisp white wine, such as Pinot Grigio, is a good accompaniment to this dish.

Prepare pasta according to package directions, cooking until tender but firm. While pasta is cooking, sauté onion in oil in heavy saucepan over medium heat, stirring occasionally, for about 4 minutes or until translucent. Add garlic and cook for 1 minute. Blend in flour. Gradually add milk and cook, stirring constantly, for about 4 minutes or until sauce is smooth and bubbly. Add spinach, ricotta cheese, ⅓ cup Parmesan cheese, tomatoes, basil, nutmeg and cayenne pepper. Season with salt and black pepper. Simmer, stirring occasionally, for about 5 minutes or until thoroughly heated. Drain pasta and place on platter. Spoon sauce on pasta and sprinkle with green onion, pine nuts and black pepper. Sprinkle individual servings with Parmesan cheese.

Serves 4.

1 16-ounce package linguine pasta
1 medium onion, chopped
3 tablespoons olive oil
3 large cloves garlic, minced
1 tablespoon all-purpose flour
2 cups milk (not 2% or skim)
1 10-ounce package frozen chopped spinach, thawed and squeezed dry
1 cup ricotta cheese
¼ cup freshly grated Parmesan cheese
10 oil-packed sun-dried tomatoes, drained and cut in thin strips
3 tablespoons chopped fresh basil or 2 teaspoons dried basil, crushed
¼ teaspoon nutmeg
¼ teaspoon cayenne pepper
   Salt and black pepper to taste
⅓ cup minced green onion
⅓ cup toasted pine nuts
   Coarsely ground black pepper
   Freshly grated Parmesan cheese

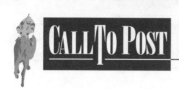

ZITI WITH TWO CHEESES, TOMATOES AND OLIVES

Havarti gives body to this pasta dish.

1½ cups chopped onion
4 large cloves garlic, minced
6 tablespoons olive oil, divided
3 28-ounce cans diced tomatoes, drained
2 tablespoons minced fresh basil or 2 teaspoons dried basil
1 teaspoon crushed red pepper flakes (or to taste)
2 cups chicken broth
   Salt and black pepper to taste
1 16-ounce package ziti pasta
2½ cups (10 ounces) firmly-packed grated Havarti cheese
⅓ cup sliced kalamata olives
½ cup (2 ounces) grated Parmesan cheese
½ cup minced basil for garnish

Sauté onion and garlic in 3 tablespoons oil in large saucepan for about 5 minutes or until onion is softened. Stir in tomatoes, 2 tablespoons basil and red pepper. Add broth. Bring to a boil, reduce heat to medium and simmer for about 1 hour or until sauce is thickened and reduce to 6 to 7 cups. Season with salt and black pepper. Prepare pasta according to package directions, cooking until tender but firm. Drain well and return to cooking pot. Add remaining 3 tablespoons oil and toss to coat evenly. Pour sauce over pasta and mix well. Stir in Havarti cheese. Spread pasta mixture in 13x9x2-inch baking dish. Sprinkle with olives and Parmesan cheese. Bake at 375° for about 30 minutes or until thoroughly heated. Sprinkle with ½ cup basil.

Serves 4 to 6.

LEMON AND HERB FLAVORED NOODLES

Delicate flavor of noodles provides a change of pace from rice and potatoes.

1 8-ounce package wide egg noodles
2 tablespoons butter, softened
2 tablespoons coarsely chopped parsley
2 tablespoons minced chives
1½ teaspoons grated lemon zest
¼ teaspoon salt
⅛ teaspoon freshly ground black pepper

Prepare noodles according to package directions, cooking until tender but firm. Drain and place in bowl. Add butter, parsley, chives, lemon zest, salt and black pepper, tossing to coat evenly. Serve immediately or keep warm until ready to serve.

Serves 4.

GARDEN PASTA

A perfect way to enjoy your garden's bounty.

Prepare pasta according to package directions, cooking until tender but firm. While pasta is cooking, blanch asparagus, broccoli, carrots and green beans in boiling water for 3 to 4 minutes and drain. Blanch zucchini in boiling water for 1 minute and drain. Sauté onion in oil in large skillet over medium-low heat until tender. Add garlic and sauté for 1 minute. Stir in tomatoes, asparagus, broccoli, carrots and green beans. Sauté for about 3 minutes. Add cream, broth, salt and black pepper. Drain pasta and add to sauce, tossing gently. Add Parmesan cheese, basil and pine nuts to vegetable sauce.

Serves 4 to 6.

1   **10-ounce package radiatore or fusilli pasta**
1   **pound asparagus, trimmed and cut in 1-inch pieces**
2   **cups small broccoli flowerets**
1   **cup julienne-cut carrots**
1   **cup diagonally-cut fresh green beans**
    Boiling water
2   **medium zucchini, cubed**
1   **medium purple onion, chopped**
¼   **cup olive oil**
3   **cloves garlic, minced**
4   **large tomatoes, peeled, seeded and chopped (about 4 cups)**
1¼   **cups whipping cream**
¾   **cup chicken broth**
¼   **teaspoon salt**
¼   **teaspoon freshly ground black pepper**
1   **cup (4 ounces) freshly grated Parmesan cheese**
1   **cup chopped fresh basil**
½   **cup pine nuts, toasted (optional)**

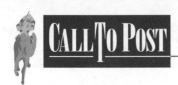

BLUE CHEESE AND FUSILLI

A contemporary twist to the classic macaroni and cheese.

1   16-ounce package fusilli pasta
3   red bell peppers, chopped
3½ cups chopped celery
2   tablespoons unsalted butter
1½ cups whipping cream
1½ cups half and half
1   pound crumbled blue cheese
1½ teaspoons celery seed
⅛   teaspoon cayenne pepper or
    to taste
    Salt and black pepper to taste
3   egg yolks, lightly beaten
½   cup chopped celery leaves
¾   cup (3 ounces) freshly grated
    Parmesan cheese

Prepare pasta according to package directions, cooking until tender but firm. While pasta is cooking, sauté bell pepper and celery in butter in large heavy skillet over medium heat for 5 to 7 minutes or just until vegetables are tender. Remove from heat and set aside. Combine cream, half and half and blue cheese in medium saucepan. Cook over low heat, stirring, until cheese is melted. Add celery seed, cayenne pepper, salt and black pepper. Remove from heat. Gradually whisk ½ of cheese mixture into beaten eggs, then add egg mixture to remaining cheese sauce in pan. Stir in celery leaves. Drain pasta and blend with cheese sauce. Spread in greased 4-quart casserole and sprinkle with Parmesan cheese. Bake at 400° for 25 to 30 minutes or until hot, bubbly and lightly browned.

Serves 10 to 12.

●

PARSLEY NOODLES

Serve with a hearty beef, veal or lamb stew.

1   12-ounce package wide egg
    noodles
2   tablespoons unsalted butter
4   teaspoons fresh lemon juice
2   teaspoons Worcestershire
    sauce
½   cup minced parsley
½   teaspoon salt
¼   teaspoon freshly ground
    black pepper

Prepare noodles according to package directions, cooking until tender but firm. Drain well and place in bowl. Add butter, lemon juice, Worcestershire sauce, parsley, salt and black pepper, tossing to coat evenly.

Serves 6.

BLUEGRASS SPICY RICE AND CHICKEN

Instant rice reduces cooking time and helps keep chicken moist. Great for kids.

Sauté garlic in oil in large skillet over medium heat for 30 seconds. Add chicken and sauté for 3 to 4 minutes or until opaque. Remove chicken and set aside. Sauté bell pepper and green onion in same skillet until softened. Season with salt, black pepper, basil and red pepper flakes. Stir in rice and cook for 1 minute. Coarsely chop tomatoes. Add tomatoes, reserved juice and broth or water combined to equal 2 cups to rice mixture. Bring to a boil. Quickly stir in picante sauce or salsa and chicken. Remove from heat, cover and let stand for 5 minutes or until liquid is absorbed. Fluff rice with fork.

Serves 4 to 6.

4   cloves garlic, minced
2   tablespoons vegetable oil
1   pound boneless, skinless chicken breast, cut in 1-inch cubes
1   medium red bell pepper, chopped
5   green onions, trimmed and chopped
   Salt and black pepper to taste
1   teaspoon dried basil, crushed
¼   teaspoon red pepper flakes (optional)
2   cups uncooked instant rice
1   14½-ounce can whole tomatoes, drained and juice reserved
   Chicken broth or water to measure 2 cups when added to reserved tomato juice
3   tablespoons picante sauce or salsa

BAKED RICE DELUXE

Cook rice in heavy skillet over medium heat, stirring constantly, until golden. Pour rice into greased 1-quart casserole. Sauté mushrooms, celery and onion in ¼ cup butter in skillet until translucent. Stir in broth and bring to a boil. Add vegetables and liquid to rice. Bake, covered, at 350° for 35 minutes or until liquid is absorbed. Stir remaining ¼ cup butter into rice mixture and fluff with fork.

Serves 6 to 8.

1   cup uncooked long grain rice
½   pound fresh mushrooms, sliced
1   cup chopped celery
½   cup chopped onion
½   cup unsalted butter, divided
2½   cups chicken broth
½   teaspoon salt
¾   teaspoon black pepper

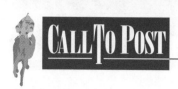

DERBY LEMON-MINT RISOTTO

Terrific as a first course or accompaniment to lamb.
If asparagus is not available, substitute 1 cup of frozen peas.

3   yellow bell peppers, seeded
    and cut in 1-inch pieces
¼   cup plus 2 tablespoons water
5   cups chicken broth, fat
    skimmed
¾   pound asparagus, trimmed
    and diagonally cut in 1½-inch
    pieces, or 1 cup peas
    Boiling salted water
6   sprigs mint
6   sprigs flat-leaf parsley
1   sprig rosemary
1   cup minced shallots
1   cup minced fennel
3   large cloves garlic, minced
1   tablespoon olive oil
1¼ cups uncooked Arborio rice
½   teaspoon ground coriander
½   cup dry white wine
2   teaspoons lemon zest
¼   cup (1 ounce) freshly grated
    Parmesan cheese
1   teaspoon salt
⅛   teaspoon freshly ground
    black pepper
3   tablespoons finely chopped
    mint, divided
4   tablespoons finely chopped
    parsley
2   teaspoons lemon juice

Combine bell pepper, water and ¼ cup broth in small saucepan. Cook over medium-low heat, stirring frequently, for 25 to 30 minutes or until peppers are very soft. Remove from heat. Purée with cooking liquid in food processor. Strain through coarse sieve and set aside. Add asparagus to boiling salted water and cook for 1 to 2 minutes or until bright green and slightly crunchy. Remove with slotted spoon, plunge into ice bath, let stand for several minutes, drain and set aside. Combine remaining 4¾ cups broth and sprigs of mint, parsley and rosemary. Bring to a boil, reduce heat and maintain at very low simmer. Sauté shallots, fennel and garlic in oil in large heavy saucepan over medium heat, stirring frequently, for about 6 minutes or until very soft but not browned. Stir in rice and coriander. Cook, stirring constantly, for about 3 minutes or until edges of rice are translucent. Add wine and lemon zest. Cook, stirring constantly, for about 30 seconds or until nearly all of wine is absorbed. Using tongs or slotted spoon, remove herb sprigs from broth. Add salt, black pepper and about ½ cup of simmering broth to rice. Cook over medium-high heat, stirring constantly, until nearly all of liquid is absorbed. Add broth, about ½ cup at a time, stirring constantly and allowing each addition to be nearly absorbed before adding next;

(Continued on next page)

(Derby Lemon-Mint Risotto, continued)

additions should take 15 to 20 minutes. Rice should be creamy-looking and each grain tender but still firm in center. Remove pan from heat and stir in pepper purée, asparagus, Parmesan cheese, 1 tablespoon chopped mint, all the chopped parsley and lemon juice. Adjust seasoning with salt and black pepper. Garnish individual servings of risotto with remaining 2 tablespoons mint. Serve immediately.

Serves 6.

ISLAND CONFETTI RICE

Melt butter in large skillet. Add rice, oranges, pineapple, almonds, bell pepper, ½ cup green onion, coconut, chutney and ginger. Cook over medium heat, stirring constantly, for about 5 minutes or until thoroughly heated. Garnish with green onion tops.

Serves 4.

1	tablespoon unsalted butter
2	cups hot cooked rice
1	11-ounce can mandarin oranges, drained and chopped
1	8-ounce can pineapple tidbits, drained
½	cup sliced almonds, toasted
¼	cup chopped red bell pepper
¼	cup chopped yellow bell pepper
½	cup chopped green onion
¼	cup chopped green onion tops for garnish
¼	cup flaked coconut, toasted
3	tablespoons hot mango chutney
¼	teaspoon ground ginger

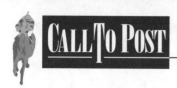
MUSHROOM RISOTTO WITH SPINACH

1 cup dried porcini, chanterelle or morel wild mushrooms or 1 cup white mushrooms, sliced

¾ cup warm chicken broth or water

¼ cup unsalted butter, divided

¼ cup olive oil, divided
Salt and freshly ground black pepper to taste

⅔ cup minced shallots

1 medium onion, minced

1½ cups uncooked Arborio rice

½ cup dry white wine

3 cloves garlic, minced

5 to 6 cups chicken broth

1 cup chopped fresh spinach

1 cup (4 ounces) freshly grated Parmesan cheese

If using wild mushrooms, rehydrate in warm broth or water. Reserve liquid and coarsely chop mushrooms. Sauté mushrooms in 2 tablespoons butter and 2 tablespoons oil in small skillet for about 3 minutes. Season with salt and black pepper and set aside. Sauté shallots and onion in remaining 2 tablespoons butter and 2 tablespoons oil in large saucepan or large deep skillet over medium heat for about 5 minutes or until translucent. Stir in rice and cook over medium heat until translucent. Stir in sherry and garlic. Cook until all liquid is absorbed. Add reserved mushroom liquid and broth, 1 cup at a time, while stirring continuously; allow liquid to be absorbed before adding next cup. With final cup, stir in spinach. Risotto should be firm to the bite but creamy. Remove from heat. Add mushrooms and Parmesan cheese. Season with salt and black pepper. **Note:** Although white mushrooms can be used, the wild mushrooms provide a richer flavor.

Serves 4 to 6.

SUMMER RISOTTO

An incredibly light entrée served with crusty bread and salad.

Blanch carrots in boiling water for 1 minute, drain, rinse with cold water and set aside. Thoroughly heat broth in saucepan and keep at simmer until ready to use. Sauté garlic and shallot in 1 tablespoon butter in large skillet over medium-high heat for 2 minutes, stirring constantly. Add rice and cook for 5 minutes or until translucent. Reduce heat to medium. Add warm broth, ½ cup at a time, while stirring continuously; allow liquid to be absorbed before adding next ½ cup. Stir in salt and black pepper. Set aside. Sauté onion in remaining 1 tablespoon butter in skillet over medium-high heat until lightly browned. Add carrots, zucchini and squash. Cook, stirring constantly, for about 5 minutes or until tender. Add arugula and cook for 1 minute. Stir vegetables into rice mixture. Add basil and oregano and sprinkle with walnuts, blue cheese and oregano sprigs.

Serves 4 to 6.

¼ cup julienne-cut carrots
Boiling water
4½ cups reduced-sodium fat-free chicken broth
2 cloves garlic, minced
2 shallots, minced
2 tablespoons butter, divided
1¼ cups uncooked Arborio rice
¼ teaspoon salt
¼ teaspoon black pepper
¼ cup thinly sliced purple onion
¼ cup thinly sliced zucchini
¼ cup thinly sliced yellow squash
¼ cup arugula
3 tablespoons chopped fresh basil
2 tablespoons chopped fresh oregano
3 tablespoons chopped walnuts, toasted
⅓ cup (1⅓ ounces) crumbled blue cheese
Fresh oregano sprigs

BROWN RICE WITH PECANS AND CHERRIES

A tart and crunchy side dish.

Sauté onion and celery in butter in large skillet over medium-low heat until softened. Add brown rice and heat thoroughly. Remove from heat and stir in cherries, pecans and onion. Season with salt and black pepper.

Serves 8.

1 medium onion, chopped
1½ cups chopped celery
6 tablespoons unsalted butter
4 cups cooked brown rice
¾ cup dried red cherries
½ cup chopped pecans, toasted
4 green onions, chopped
Salt and black pepper to taste

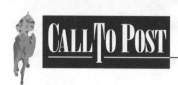

CURRIED PILAF

Delicious with pork tenderloin.

1 medium onion, diced
¼ cup unsalted butter
2 teaspoons curry powder
1 cup uncooked long grain rice
2 cups chicken broth
¼ cup pine nuts, toasted
2 tablespoons minced chives
  Salt and black pepper to taste

Sauté onion in butter in large saucepan over low heat for 5 minutes or until softened. Add curry powder and rice. Cook over medium heat, stirring to prevent sticking, for 5 minutes. Stir in broth and bring to a boil. Simmer, covered, for 20 to 25 minutes or until liquid is absorbed. Add pine nuts, chives, salt and black pepper. Fluff with fork.

Serves 6.

FIESTA RICE

Dish can be assembled several hours in advance and stored in refrigerator. Bring to room temperature before baking.

4 cloves garlic, minced
1 large onion, chopped
½ cup butter
4 cups cooked white rice
1 cup regular or low-fat cottage cheese
2 cups regular or low-fat sour cream
1 tablespoon Worcestershire sauce
2 bay leaves, crumbled
1¼ teaspoons Beau Monde seasoning
½ teaspoon salt
½ teaspoon black pepper
1½ cups (6 ounces) shredded Cheddar cheese
1½ cups (6 ounces) shredded Monterey Jack cheese
2 4½-ounce cans diced green chilies
3 cups grated zucchini, blotted very dry

Sauté garlic and onion in butter in large skillet over low heat until translucent. Remove from heat. Add rice, cottage cheese, sour cream, Worcestershire sauce, bay leaves, beau monde seasoning, salt and black pepper to garlic and onion, blending well. Combine Cheddar cheese and Monterey Jack cheese. In greased 4-quart casserole, in order listed, layer: ⅓ rice mixture, ½ chilies, ½ zucchini and 1 cup mixed cheeses. Repeat layers, add remaining rice and top with remaining 1 cup cheese. Bake, uncovered, at 375° for 30 minutes or until bubbly and thoroughly heated.

Serves 8 to 10.

COUSCOUS WITH PINE NUTS AND MINT

A unique addition to roasted chicken.

2   14½-ounce cans chicken broth
6   tablespoons butter
3   cups couscous
½   cup dried currants
½   cup pine nuts, toasted
5   green onions, thinly sliced
½   cup minced mint
2   tablespoons minced fresh dill
    Salt and black pepper to taste

Combine broth and butter in saucepan. Bring to a boil, remove from heat and stir in couscous. Let stand, covered, for 5 minutes. Fluff couscous with fork and spoon into bowl. Stir in currants, pine nuts, onion, mint and dill. Season with salt and black pepper.

Serves 8.

BARLEY RISOTTO WITH CHICKEN

To add color, garnish with additional red onion rings, julienned carrots and parsley.

Sauté carrot and thyme in oil in Dutch oven over medium-high heat for 1 minute. Add celery, leek and onion and sauté for 1 minute. Stir in salt, black pepper and chicken and sauté for 5 minutes. Add barley and sauté for 1 minute. Add broth and water to chicken mixture, bring to a boil, reduce heat and simmer, covered, for 40 minutes. Remove from heat. Discard thyme sprig and stir in parsley and cheese.

Serves 6 to 8.

1   cup finely diced carrots
1   tablespoon chopped fresh thyme or 1 teaspoon dried thyme
1   tablespoon olive oil
¾   cup diced celery
¾   cup leek, cleaned and thinly sliced
½   cup minced onion
½   teaspoon salt
¼   teaspoon black pepper
6   chicken breast halves, skin and bone removed and cut in ¼-inch strips
1¾ cup uncooked pearl barley
6   cups chicken broth
1   cup water
½   cup chopped parsley
¼   cup (1 ounce) freshly grated Parmesan cheese

131

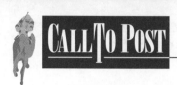

COUSCOUS WITH VEGETABLES AND FETA CHEESE

Vegetable mixture can be prepared a day in advance and stored, covered, in refrigerator. Reheat before adding to couscous.

½   cup chopped red onion
4   large cloves garlic, minced
2   tablespoons olive oil
4   red-skinned potatoes, cut in ½-inch cubes
3   carrots, diagonally cut in ½-inch slices
2   small zucchini, cut in ½-inch slices
1   tablespoon chili powder
⅛   to ¼ teaspoon ground cinnamon
½   teaspoon ground cumin
1   teaspoon curry powder
1   teaspoon paprika
½   teaspoon turmeric
1   15-ounce can tomato sauce
½   cup water
    Salt and black pepper to taste
1   10-ounce package couscous
1   cup (4 ounces) crumbled feta cheese

Sauté onion and garlic in oil in heavy skillet over medium-high heat for about 4 minutes or until tender. Add potatoes and carrots and sauté for 5 minutes. Stir in zucchini, chili powder, cinnamon, cumin, curry powder, paprika and turmeric. Cook for 1 minute or until spices are fragrant. Add tomato sauce and water. Bring to a boil, reduce heat and simmer, covered, for about 10 minutes. Remove cover and simmer for about 10 minutes or until potatoes are tender and sauce is slightly thickened. Season with salt and black pepper. Prepare couscous according to package directions. Pour into large bowl, add hot vegetable mixture and sprinkle with feta cheese.

Serves 8.

NUTTY WILD RICE PILAF

Pilaf is a good accompaniment with pork or poultry.

Sauté wild rice and onion in butter in large skillet over medium heat for 5 minutes. Add broth, bring to a boil, reduce heat and simmer, covered, for 25 minutes. Stir in white rice and rosemary. Cook, covered, for 15 to 20 minutes or until rice is tender. Add walnuts, parsley, salt and black pepper.

Serves 6.

¾   cup uncooked wild rice, rinsed and well drained
3   green onions, chopped
3   tablespoons butter
4   cups chicken broth
½   cup uncooked long grain white rice
½   teaspoon dried rosemary
½   cup walnuts or pecans, toasted
½   cup minced parsley
    Salt and black pepper to taste

FISH & SEAFOOD

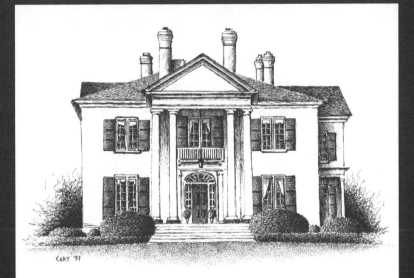

For three generations, Claiborne Farm has been one of the world's leading Thoroughbred farms. Managed since 1972 by Seth Hancock, the grandson of the farm's founders A. B. and Nancy Clay Hancock, Claiborne has raised many of racing's greatest champions, including Horse of the Year Forego, Claiborne's Kentucky Derby winner Swale and the undefeated filly champion Personal Ensign.

As a commercial stallion operation, sires standing at Claiborne — such as Bold Ruler, Nijinsky II, Mr. Prospector and Danzig — have dominated the leading sires list for decades.

An important part of American racing history, Claiborne's sire roster once included America's most popular racehorse, Secretariat, who is buried in the farm's cemetery.

Claiborne

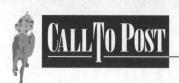

Fish & Seafood

DEVILED CRAB

Combine crabmeat, eggs, onion and parsley. Add mayonnaise, sherry, lemon juice, mustard and Worcestershire sauce, mixing lightly but thoroughly. Combine bread crumbs and butter. Add ½ of crumbs to crabmeat mixture. Spread in 1½-quart casserole and top with remaining crumbs. Bake at 350° until lightly browned. **Note:** Individual shells can be used instead of casserole.

Serves 4.

2 cups crabmeat
2 hard-cooked eggs, chopped
1 teaspoon grated onion
1 teaspoon minced parsley
1 cup mayonnaise
3 tablespoons sherry
2 teaspoons lemon juice
½ teaspoon prepared mustard
½ teaspoon Worcestershire sauce
1 cup bread crumbs
1 cup butter, melted

CAJUN SHRIMP WITH RICE

A great do-ahead dish.

Sauté onion, green onion, garlic and celery in butter in large skillet until tender. Stir in flour and cook until lightly browned. Add water, tomato puree, bay leaves, Worcestershire sauce, hot pepper sauce, sugar, salt, black pepper and thyme. Simmer, uncovered, for 25 minutes, stirring occasionally. Add shrimp and cook just until shrimp are done. **Note:** Serve shrimp with sauce on rice. Sauce can be prepared a day in advance and stored in refrigerator. Reheat and add shrimp.

Serves 4 to 6.

1 medium onion, chopped
2 green onions, chopped
3 or 4 cloves garlic, minced
¼ cup chopped celery
½ cup butter
2 tablespoons all-purpose flour
2½ cups water
1 10½-ounce can tomato puree
2 bay leaves
1 tablespoon Worcestershire sauce
4 drops hot pepper sauce
½ teaspoon sugar
1 teaspoon salt
⅛ teaspoon black pepper
½ teaspoon thyme
1 pound fresh shrimp, peeled and deveined

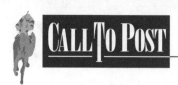

SEAFOOD KABOB

¼ cup teriyaki sauce
2 tablespoons lime juice
1 teaspoon vegetable oil
2 tablespoons honey mustard
1 clove garlic, crushed
1½ pounds shrimp
1½ pounds sea scallops

Combine teriyaki sauce, lime juice, oil, mustard and garlic, blending well. Add shrimp and scallops to marinade, turning to coat on all sides. Chill, covered, for 2 to 4 hours, stirring occasionally. Thread shrimp and scallops on skewers. Grill over medium-hot coals for 4 to 6 minutes, basting occasionally with remaining marinade. **Note:** Serve kabob with rice pilaf.

Serves 4.

BAKED SHRIMP

1 cup butter, melted
¼ cup dry white wine
¼ cup fresh minced parsley
2 tablespoons fresh lemon juice
3 large cloves garlic, minced
2 teaspoons dried basil
1 teaspoon Worcestershire sauce
¾ to 1 teaspoon hot pepper sauce
½ teaspoon salt
2 pounds large fresh shrimp (about 32), peeled with tails left intact and deveined
½ cup dry unseasoned bread crumbs

Combine butter, wine, parsley, lemon juice, garlic, basil, Worcestershire sauce, hot pepper sauce and salt in shallow 2-quart casserole. Set aside ¼ cup of mixture. Place shrimp in sauce, mixing thoroughly. Combine bread crumbs with reserved sauce and sprinkle over shrimp. Bake at 450° for 10 to 15 minutes. Serve immediately.

Serves 6 to 8.

SHRIMP SAUTÉ

Place tomatoes in colander, sprinkle with salt and let drain in sink for 30 to 60 minutes. Sauté zucchini, seasoned with salt and black pepper, in 2 tablespoons oil in heavy medium skillet over medium-high heat until browned. Add bell pepper and cook, stirring gently, for 1 minute. Remove from heat and set aside. Heat remaining 3 tablespoons oil with chili pepper in large heavy skillet over high heat until pepper is darkened; remove and discard. Add shrimp, sliced garlic and thyme sprig to seasoned oil. Sauté, shaking pan constantly, until shrimp become bright pink. Season with salt and black pepper. Discard garlic if it has burned. Add tomatoes and cook for 2 to 3 minutes or until excess liquid has evaporated. Add zucchini mixture, parsley, minced garlic and thyme. Check seasoning. Remove from heat and garnish with lemon wedges. Serve from skillet, accompanied by French bread.

Serves 4.

8 to 10 Italian plum tomatoes, peeled, quartered and seeded
Salt
1 medium zucchini, finely diced
Freshly ground black pepper
5 tablespoons olive oil, divided
1 red bell pepper, roasted, peeled and finely sliced
1 small dried hot chili pepper, crumbled
1 pound fresh shrimp, peeled and deveined
2 large cloves garlic, finely sliced
1 large sprig fresh thyme
3 tablespoons finely minced fresh parsley
2 cloves garlic, finely minced
2 tablespoons finely minced fresh thyme
Lemon wedges for garnish
French bread

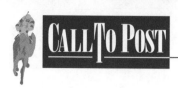

POOR MAN'S LOBSTER

Easy, company will beg for more.

2	pounds unpeeled fresh shrimp
½	cup margarine, melted
1	cup olive oil
¼	cup soy sauce
¼	cup lemon juice
4	cloves garlic, crushed
1⅓	tablespoons Italian seasoning

Place shrimp in shallow baking dish. Combine margarine, oil, soy sauce, lemon juice, garlic and Italian seasoning. Pour over shrimp. Bake at 350° for 30 minutes or until shrimp are done. Serve in soup bowls with French bread slices for dipping in sauce. **Variation:** Sprinkle 1 tablespoon of freshly ground black pepper over shrimp before baking.

Serves 6.

CAROLINA SHRIMP AND GRITS

Satisfying!

GRITS

4	cups water
1	teaspoon salt
1	cup instant grits
½	cup butter
2	cups (8 ounces) shredded Cheddar cheese
¼	teaspoon garlic powder
3	eggs
¾	cup half and half

Combine water and salt in saucepan. Bring to a boil. Gradually add grits and cook for about 5 minutes, stirring constantly. Remove from heat and stir in butter, Cheddar cheese and garlic powder. Beat eggs and half and half together. Add to grits. Pour mixture into greased 2-quart casserole. Bake at 350° for 45 minutes.

SHRIMP

¼	cup diced onion
2	tablespoons butter, divided
21	to 26 fresh shrimp, peeled and deveined
1½	teaspoons herbes de Provence
1½	teaspoons Cajun seasoning
2	slices bacon or strips of ham, diced and cooked crisp
	Minced fresh parsley
	Lemon wedges

Sauté onion in 1 tablespoon butter in saucepan until softened. Add shrimp, herbes de Provence, Cajun seasoning and remaining 1 tablespoon butter. Cook, stirring constantly, until gray sauce forms. Pour over grits and garnish with bacon or ham, parsley and lemon.

Serves 4.

SHRIMP RÉMOULADE WITH FRIED GREEN TOMATOES

Combine onion, green onion, garlic, oil, vinegar, mustard, salt, cayenne pepper and paprika in blender container. Blend for 5 to 6 seconds. Separately chill sauce and shrimp overnight. Add shrimp to sauce. Prepare tomatoes. Roll or shake tomato slices in mixture of flour, cornmeal, salt, black pepper and paprika. Fry in small amount of vegetable oil in large skillet until tomatoes are tender, and lightly brown on both sides. Serve sauce on tomatoes.

Serves 6.

1   cup minced onion
½   cup chopped green onion
3   cloves garlic, pressed
¾   cup vegetable oil
¼   cup tarragon vinegar
½   cup brown Creole mustard
2   teaspoons salt
¾   teaspoon cayenne pepper
2   teaspoons paprika
2   pounds shrimp, peeled, deveined and boiled
    Green tomatoes, sliced ¼-inch thick; enough tomatoes to allow for 3-4 slices per portion
¼   cup all-purpose flour
¼   cup cornmeal
    Salt and black pepper to taste
    Paprika to taste
    Vegetable oil

MAHOGANY GLAZED SALMON FILETS

Combine sugar and water in saucepan. Heat, without stirring, until syrup is medium-dark caramel color. Remove from heat and add ginger and garlic. Let stand for 2 minutes. Gradually add soy sauce. Cook, stirring frequently, until sugar is dissolved. Bring to a boil, remove from heat and reserve ½ cup. Brush salmon filets with glaze 3 or 4 times over several hours; do not brush skin of fish. Place salmon, skin side down, in roasting pan. Bake at 450° for 8 to 12 minutes, depending on thickness of filets. Serve with reserved glaze.

Serves 6 to 8.

1   cup sugar
⅓   cup water
1   inch ginger root, slivered
6   cloves garlic
2   cups soy sauce
2   pounds salmon filet, skin intact and cut in 6 to 8 pieces

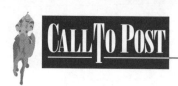

SPICY CATFISH

Terrific!

2	pounds catfish filets
	Salt to taste
2	tablespoons vegetable oil
1	cup chopped onion
1	cup chopped green bell
	pepper
1	tablespoon chopped jalapeño
	pepper
2	cloves garlic, minced
1	bay leaf, finely crushed
½	teaspoon dried oregano
½	teaspoon dried thyme
	Freshly ground black pepper
2	tablespoons olive oil
3	tablespoons ground toasted
	almonds
¼	cup minced fresh parsley
18	thin lemon slices
	Paprika

Cut catfish into 12 portions. Season with salt. Cut 6 12x12-inch squares aluminum foil, fold in halves and cut largest possible heart shape. Open hearts, brush with oil and place 1 piece catfish on right side. Sauté onion, bell pepper, jalapeño pepper, garlic, bay leaf, oregano, thyme and black pepper in olive oil in large heavy skillet over low heat for 5 minutes, stirring occasionally. Add almonds and parsley. Spoon mixture evenly on catfish on foil, top each with second filet, arrange 3 lemon slices on filet and sprinkle with paprika. Fold left side half of foil over catfish and fold edges to tightly secure. Place packets on baking sheet. Bake at 450° for 15 to 20 minutes or until foil is puffed. Make crosswise slit in length and width of each packet and fold edges back.

Serves 6.

BROILED SALMON WITH ZESTY LEMON MUSTARD

2	tablespoons coarse-grain
	mustard
2	tablespoons grated lemon
	zest
2	tablespoons fresh lemon juice
½	teaspoon salt
¼	teaspoon black pepper
1½	pounds salmon filet, cut in
	4 pieces

Combine mustard, zest, lemon juice, salt and black pepper. Place salmon, skin side down, on broiler pan. Brush with mustard sauce. Broil salmon for 6 to 8 minutes or until center is opaque. Serve immediately.

Serves 4.

SALMON WITH ARUGULA, TOMATO AND CAPER SAUCE

Combine tomatoes, arugula, basil or Italian parsley, ½ cup oil, shallots, lemon juice and capers. Season with salt and black pepper. Brush both sides of salmon with oil and season with salt and black pepper. Broil or grill skin side down, without turning, for about 4 minutes or just until cooked through. Spoon tomato mixture on individual servings of salmon and garnish with lemon wedges.

Serves 4.

1	pound plum tomatoes, seeded and chopped
¾	cup lightly-packed chopped arugula, fresh basil leaves or fresh Italian parsley
½	cup olive oil
1	shallot, chopped
1½	tablespoons fresh lemon juice
1	tablespoon drained capers
	Salt and black pepper to taste
4	6-ounce salmon filets
	Olive oil
	Lemon wedges

ORIENTAL SWORDFISH/TUNA

An easy to make entrée with a twist!

Toast sesame seeds in small dry pan over low heat until they pop. Set aside. Combine garlic, ginger, mustard and soy sauce. Using food processor or blender, process until blended. Process in vinegar. Gradually add peanut oil and sesame oil, drop by drop at first and then in stream until all oil is incorporated and sauce is emulsified. Set aside. Brush fish with peanut oil and season with salt and black pepper. Broil or grill for 3 to 4 minutes on each side or until just cooked through. Place filets on individual plates, top with sauce and sprinkle with green onion, sesame seeds and cilantro.

Serves 6.

3	tablespoons sesame seeds
2	cloves garlic
3	inch piece fresh ginger root, peeled
1½	tablespoons hot or Dijon mustard
3	tablespoons soy sauce
⅓	cup rice or white wine vinegar
⅔	cup peanut oil
¼	cup dark Oriental sesame oil
6	6-ounce swordfish or tuna filets, ¾ to 1 inch thick
	Peanut oil
	Salt and freshly ground black pepper
½	cup finely chopped green onion
¼	cup chopped fresh cilantro (optional)

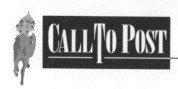

RED SNAPPER AMANDINE

6　red snapper filets
　　Salt and black pepper to taste
　　All-purpose flour
1½　cups butter, divided
1　cup sliced bleached almonds
　　Juice of 1 lemon

Season snapper with salt and black pepper. Coat lightly with flour. Sauté filets in ½ cup butter in saucepan until cooked and lightly browned. Place in baking pan. Melt remaining 1 cup butter in skillet, add almonds and cook until almonds are lightly browned. Spoon almond mixture on filets and sprinkle with lemon juice. Bake at 375° for 3 to 5 minutes or until lightly browned.

Serves 6.

GRILLED TROUT WITH HERBS

The perfect partner with a pasta salad.

2　tablespoons dried leaf
　　rosemary, divided
1　tablespoon rubbed sage
　　Salt and black pepper to taste
¼　cup olive oil
1　3½-pound lake trout or 4
　　8- to 10-ounce rainbow trout,
　　cleaned with head and tail
　　intact
1　large lime, sliced

Combine 1 tablespoon rosemary, sage and black pepper with oil. Rub herb mixture on inside and outside of trout. Place lime slices in cavity. Sprinkle remaining 1 tablespoon rosemary over hot coals. Place trout on prepared grill or on double layer of greased aluminum foil with a few holes in it. Grill for 5 to 6 minutes on each side or until fish begins to flake when tested with fork tines; baste fish during grilling. Using greased spatula, carefully transfer trout to platter.

Serves 4.

CAYMAN SNAPPER

Combine tomatoes, garlic, capers, wine and marinara sauce. Place filets in baking pan. Spoon tomato sauce over filets. Bake at 350° for 20 minutes. Garnish with lemon slices.

Serves 2.

2 fresh plum tomatoes, chopped
2 tablespoons garlic, chopped
2 teaspoons capers
1 cup white wine
1 cup marinara sauce
2 snapper filets
  Lemon slices

TROUT—BLUEGRASS STYLE

Season trout with salt and white pepper. Combine eggs and milk. Dip filets in liquid, then roll in bread crumbs. Combine butter, eggs, parsley and pimento, mixing to form paste. Using just enough oil to prevent sticking, cook filets on grill for about 5 to 6 minutes on each side or until golden. Place on warm platter. Spread butter paste on each filet and top with 2 or 3 lemon slices. Serve immediately.

Serves 6.

6 to 9 trout, cut in filets
½ teaspoon salt
½ teaspoon white pepper
3 eggs, well beaten
¼ cup milk
1½ cups fine toasted bread crumbs
½ cup butter, softened
2 hard-cooked eggs, finely chopped
⅓ cup finely chopped fresh parsley
2 tablespoons finely chopped pimento
3 tablespoons vegetable oil
2 lemons, thinly sliced

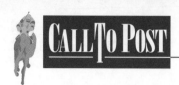

GRILLED TUNA WITH MINTED ORANGE CHUTNEY

FISH
- 1 medium orange
- 2 tablespoons lemon juice
- 1 tablespoon soy sauce
- ½ teaspoon dried thyme
- ¼ teaspoon fennel seed, crushed
- 1 large clove garlic, minced
  Freshly ground black pepper
- ¼ cup olive oil
- 4 6- to 8-ounce tuna steaks, about 1 inch thick

Prepare minted orange chutney. Finely grate peel from orange into shallow baking dish. Cut orange in half and squeeze to extract juice into baking dish. Add lemon juice, soy sauce, thyme, fennel, garlic and black pepper, mixing well. Gradually whisk in oil, blending until smooth. Add tuna to marinade, turning to coat on all sides. Marinate at room temperature for 30 to 45 minutes. Remove tuna, reserving marinade. Grill or broil steaks, 5 to 6 inches from heat source, for 6 minutes, turning once and basting frequently with reserved marinade. Serve with minted orange chutney.

MINTED ORANGE CHUTNEY
- 1 large seedless orange, peeled and finely chopped
- 1 tablespoon finely chopped red onion
- 1 tablespoon finely chopped fresh mint or 1 teaspoon dried mint
- 1 tablespoon finely chopped fresh green or red chili pepper
- 1 teaspoon orange juice
- 2 tablespoons chopped yellow bell pepper

Combine orange, onion, mint, chili pepper, orange juice and bell pepper. Chill, covered, for 30 to 60 minutes; do not prepare too far in advance of using to avoid losing freshness and texture.

Serves 4.

POULTRY

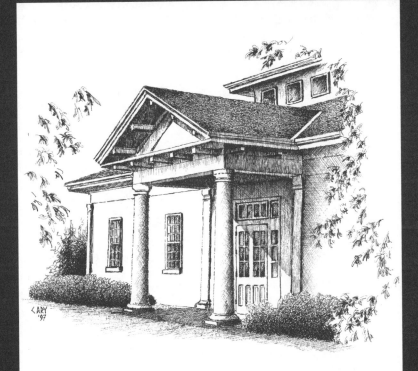

Josephine Abercrombie's Pin Oak Stud is situated on 950 acres near Versailles, Kentucky. Involved in racing since 1949, Pin Oak is recognized for their successful breeding and racing interests. Abercrombie was named the Thoroughbred Owners and Breeders Association's Breeder of the Year for 1995. Home to a small and selective group of young stallions, Pin Oak stands champions Maria's Mon, homebred Peaks And Valleys and Sky Classic, as well as graded stakes winners Caller I.D., Prospectors Gamble and Wekiva Springs.

Pin Oak Stud

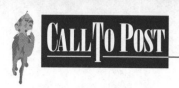

Poultry

CHICKEN ROAST WITH PINE NUT STUFFING

Rinse chicken and blot dry with paper towel. Season inside and surface of chicken with ½ teaspoon salt and ¼ teaspoon black pepper. Sauté scallions in ¼ cup butter in large saucepan over medium heat for 3 to 5 minutes. Add pine nuts and cook for 3 minutes. Stir in rice, parsley, remaining 1 teaspoon salt and ¼ teaspoon black pepper. Spoon rice mixture loosely into chicken cavity and place remainder in buttered casserole. Secure chicken legs with string and place in small roasting pan. Melt remaining 2 tablespoons butter and brush over chicken. Bake at 375° for 1¼ hours, basting at 20 minute intervals with pan liquid; juices should be clear when thigh is pierced. Bake remaining rice stuffing during final 30 minutes of roasting time.

Serves 4.

1	3 to 4-pound roasting chicken
1½	teaspoons salt, divided
½	teaspoon freshly ground black pepper, divided
4	scallions, finely chopped
¼	cup plus 2 tablespoons butter, divided
¼	cup pine nuts
3	cups cooked rice
2	tablespoons chopped parsley

CRUNCHY CAJUN CHICKEN

Combine biscuit mix, salt, Cajun or Creole seasoning, paprika and pecans. Dip chicken pieces in buttermilk, coat with dry mixture and place in greased 13x9x2-inch baking pan. Drizzle butter over chicken. Bake, uncovered, at 350° for 1 hour.

Serves 6.

1	cup buttermilk biscuit mix
½	teaspoon salt
½	teaspoon Cajun or Creole seasoning
1	teaspoon paprika
½	cup finely chopped pecans
6	chicken breast halves, skin and bone removed
½	cup buttermilk
½	cup butter, melted

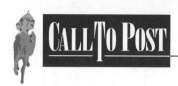

LEMON-HERB ROAST CHICKEN

½ cup butter, softened
2 tablespoons chopped fresh rosemary or 2 teaspoons dried rosemary
2 tablespoons chopped fresh thyme or 2 teaspoons dried thyme
3 large cloves garlic, minced
1½ teaspoons grated lemon peel
Salt and black pepper to taste
1 6½ to 7-pound roasting chicken
¼ cup dry white wine
1 cup chicken broth
2 tablespoons all-purpose flour
Lemon wedges
Rosemary sprigs

Combine butter, rosemary, thyme, garlic and lemon peel, stirring to blend. Season with salt and black pepper. Rinse chicken and blot dry with paper towel. Slip hand under skin over chicken breast to separate skin from meat. Reserving 2 tablespoons herb butter, rub remainder on chicken breast under skin, then on outside of chicken. Sprinkle salt and black pepper on chicken. Truss to help retain shape and place in large heavy roasting pan. Bake at 450° for 20 minutes, reduce temperature to 375° and bake for about 1¼ hours or until meat thermometer inserted in thickest part of inner thigh registers 175° and juices are clear when thigh is pierced. Transfer chicken to platter and tent with aluminum foil to keep warm. Pour pan liquid into large glass measuring cup. Skim fat. Add wine to roasting pan. Place over high heat, bring wine to a boil and scrape to dislodge browned bits. Add wine liquid to pan liquid. Add enough broth to measure 2¼ cups liquid. Melt reserved 2 tablespoons herb butter in heavy saucepan over medium-high heat. Whisk in flour until smooth and cook for about 3 minutes or until flour begins to color. Gradually whisk in liquid, bring to a boil and cook for about 7 minutes, whisking occasionally, or until thickened to sauce consistency. Season with salt and black pepper. Arrange lemon and rosemary around chicken and serve with gravy.

Serves 4.

TOMATO-HERB CHICKEN

Rinse chicken and blot dry with paper towel. Heat oil in heavy 12-inch skillet over medium-high heat. Arrange chicken pieces skin side down and without pieces touching in skillet. Brown over medium or lower heat for about 15 minutes or until rich amber color, season with salt and black pepper, turning with two wooden spatulas. Remove chicken to platter. Retain 2 tablespoons chicken fat in skillet. Sauté carrot, onion, 3 table-spoons parsley and sage for 8 minutes or until onion begins to turn yellow. Stir in lemon zest and sauté, stirring often, for 3 minutes or until onion is deep golden; do not burn glaze. Blend in garlic, ground cloves, tomatoes and water, scraping to loosen glaze from bottom of pan. Add chicken and 2 tablespoons lemon juice. Cook, cov-ered, for 15 minutes; remove cover and cook for additional 10 minutes, turning chicken to moisten. Sauce should be thick and cling to chicken. Sprinkle remaining 3 to 4 tablespoons lemon juice over chicken and check salt and black pepper seasoning. Place chicken on warm platter, spooning pan juices over pieces. Sprinkle with parsley.

Serves 4 to 6.

1 3½-pound frying or roasting chicken, cut in 8 pieces
3 tablespoons extra-virgin olive oil
  Salt and freshly ground black pepper to taste
½ small carrot, minced
½ medium onion, minced
¼ cup plus 1 tablespoon minced Italian parsley, divided
8 fresh or dried whole sage leaves
  Zest of 1 large lemon
1 large clove garlic, minced
  Pinch of ground cloves
¾ cup peeled, seeded and chopped ripe tomatoes or chopped canned tomatoes, drained
⅔ cup water or liquid from canned tomatoes
5 to 6 tablespoons fresh lemon juice, divided

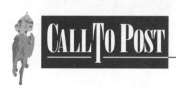
CHICKEN CORTONA

¼ pound large green olives, pitted
¼ pound Kalamata olives, pitted
Boiling water
1 3½ to 4 pound chicken
½ teaspoon salt
½ teaspoon freshly ground black pepper
2 teaspoons herbes de Provence, divided
2 tablespoons olive oil
1½ tablespoons extra-virgin olive oil
2 large heads garlic, separated into cloves and peeled
2 plum tomatoes, peeled, seeded and chopped, or 1 cup drained chopped canned tomatoes
1 tablespoon sherry wine vinegar
¾ cup dry white wine
2 cups chicken broth
1 tablespoon lemon juice
¼ cup chopped parsley

Add olives to medium saucepan of boiling water and cook for 1 minute. Drain, rinse under cold running water and set aside. Rinse chicken and blot dry with paper towel. Cut into pieces, separating legs and thighs, wings and cutting breast halves crosswise to make 10 pieces. Trim all excess fat. Season with salt, black pepper and 1 teaspoon herbes de Provence. Cook ½ of chicken in 2 tablespoons olive oil in large flameproof casserole over medium high heat for 8 to 10 minutes, turning to lightly brown on all sides. Remove chicken to platter and repeat with remaining pieces. Pour fat from pan. Pour extra-virgin olive oil into pan and place over medium heat. Sauté garlic for 1 to 2 minutes or until it begins to turn golden. Add tomatoes and remaining 1 teaspoon herbes de Provence. Increase heat to medium high and cook, stirring often, for 2 to 3 minutes or until tomatoes are softened and some of liquid is slightly thickened. Stir in vinegar and cook for 30 seconds. Add wine, bring to a boil and cook for 1 to 2 minutes or until liquid is reduced by ⅓. Place chicken in pan and add broth. Simmer, covered, for 20 minutes. Add olives and lemon juice. Simmer, partially covered, for 15 minutes or until chicken is tender. Season with salt and black pepper to taste. Remove from heat

(Continued on next page)

(Chicken Cortona, continued)

and let stand, covered, for about 10 minutes. Garnish with parsley. **Note:** Flavors mellow if reheated and served the following day. Dish can be frozen for up to 3 months; to freshen, stir 1 crushed clove garlic and 1 tea-spoon lemon juice into thawed dish and simmer for 1 to 2 minutes before serving.

Serves 4 to 6.

MUSTARD CHICKEN
A great do-ahead dish.

Cut chicken breasts crosswise in halves. Trim and discard fat from all chicken pieces. Sauté onion in butter in large flameproof casserole over medium heat, stirring occasionally, for about 3 minutes or until soft and translucent. Add chicken and cook, turning, for 5 to 7 minutes or until no longer pink on outside. Whisk Dijon mustard, honey mustard and Pommery mustard together in small bowl. Gradually whisk in wine. Pour mixture over chicken. Bring to a boil, add broth, reduce heat and simmer, partially covered, for 25 to 30 minutes or until chicken is tender and juicy with no trace of pink. Remove from heat and stir in sour cream. **Note:** Dish can be frozen for up to 3 months. If sauce appears separated after reheat-ing, remove chicken, whisk sauce briefly to recombine and serve.

Serves 6.

2	**pounds chicken breast halves, skin and bone removed**
1	**pound chicken thighs, skin and bone removed**
1	**medium onion, minced**
2	**tablespoons butter**
¼	**cup imported Dijon mustard**
3	**tablespoons honey mustard**
2	**tablespoons Pommery (coarse grainy) mustard**
¾	**cup Chardonnay wine**
1½	**cups fresh chicken broth or low-sodium canned broth**
⅓	**cup sour cream**

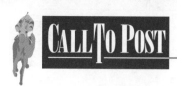

CHICKEN AND ASPARAGUS IN GINGER SAUCE

4   chicken breast halves, skin
    and bone removed
2   large green onions with tops,
    minced
3   tablespoons soy sauce
¼   cup rice wine, divided
2   tablespoons sesame oil,
    divided
1   tablespoon chopped peeled
    ginger root
½   teaspoon minced garlic
2   tablespoons firmly-packed
    brown sugar
½   teaspoon hot chili oil
1   teaspoon finely grated orange
    zest
½   teaspoon finely grated lemon
    zest
¾   cup chicken broth, divided
1   teaspoon cornstarch
1½ pounds thin stalks asparagus,
    trimmed and cut in 2-inch
    pieces
2   green onions, cut in julienne
    strips
3   cups cooked white rice
    Orange zest

Combine chicken, green onions, soy sauce, 2 tablespoons rice wine, 1 table-spoon sesame oil, ginger, garlic, brown sugar, chili oil, orange zest and lemon zest in shallow dish. Chill, tightly covered, for 4 hours, stirring occasionally. Combine ½ cup broth, remaining 2 tablespoons wine and cornstarch, blending until smooth. Heat remaining 1 tablespoon sesame oil in large non-stick skillet over high heat. Add chicken mixture and cook until chicken is opaque. Using slotted spoon, transfer chicken to bowl. Add remaining ¼ cup broth and asparagus to liquid in skillet. Reduce heat to medium-low and cook, covered, for about 3 minutes or just until aspara-gus is tender. Blend in cornstarch mixture and add cooked chicken to asparagus. Stir and cook for about 2 minutes or until sauce is translucent. Stir in green onion strips. Mound cooked rice in individual serving bowls and top with chicken mixture. Garnish with orange zest.

Serves 4.

FETA CHICKEN WITH MUSHROOMS AND TOMATOES

Combine ½ cup feta cheese, green onion and black pepper. Using smooth side of mallet, lightly pound chicken breasts to flatten. Divide cheese filling among chicken pieces, carefully fold chicken around filling and place in shallow baking dish. Bake at 350° for 35 to 40 minutes. While chicken is baking, sauté shallots, garlic, mushrooms, parsley or basil and oregano in butter in skillet for 2 to 3 minutes. Blend in flour. Gradually add wine, stirring constantly until well blended and slightly thickened. Stir in broth. Add tomatoes and 1 tablespoon feta cheese. Simmer for 10 minutes. Check seasonings. Serve sauce over chicken.

Serves 4.

½ cup (2 ounces) feta cheese plus 1 tablespoon feta cheese, divided
¼ cup minced green onion
Freshly ground black pepper to taste
4 chicken breast halves, skin and bone removed
2 small shallots, minced
3 small cloves garlic, minced
1 cup sliced mushrooms
2 tablespoons fresh parsley or fresh basil or 2 teaspoons dried parsley or basil
1 teaspoon oregano
3 tablespoons butter
1 tablespoon all-purpose flour
⅓ cup white wine
½ cup chicken broth
½ cup diced red tomatoes

HOORAY POULET SAUTÉ

Season chicken with salt and black pepper. Sauté pieces in butter in large skillet, turning to brown on both sides. Remove chicken from skillet and set aside. Cook scallions in pan drippings for 2 minutes; do not brown. Add wine and cook to reduce liquid by ½. Blend in flour. Gradually whisk in broth, mustard and brown bouquet sauce. Stir in tarragon. Return chicken to skillet. Cook, covered, for 15 minutes over low heat. Turn chicken and cook, uncovered, for 10 additional minutes. Add lemon juice. Sprinkle with parsley.

Serves 4.

4 chicken breast halves, skin and bone removed
Salt and black pepper to taste
2 tablespoons butter
1 bunch scallions, chopped
½ cup dry white wine
2 tablespoons all-purpose flour
1 cup chicken broth
1 teaspoon Dijon mustard
½ teaspoon brown bouquet sauce
1 teaspoon dried tarragon
½ teaspoon lemon juice
Chopped parsley

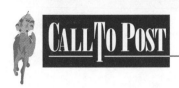

HONEY DIJON CHICKEN

A wonderful outdoor barbecue dish.

½ cup raspberry vinegar
2 tablespoons soy sauce
2 tablespoons honey
1½ tablespoons Dijon mustard
Freshly ground black pepper
to taste
2 tablespoons minced fresh
basil or 2 teaspoons dried
½ teaspoon dried thyme
4 chicken breast halves, skin
and bone removed

Combine vinegar, soy sauce, honey, mustard, black pepper, basil and thyme in shallow baking dish. Add chicken and turn to coat thoroughly. Marinate at room temperature for 15 minutes. Reserving marinade, grill chicken over medium coals for about 4 minutes on each side or until thoroughly cooked. Place on platter and tent with aluminum foil to keep warm. Pour marinade into small saucepan, bring to a boil and cook to reduce liquid by ½. Pour over chicken.

Serves 4.

CHICKEN WITH LEMON CREAM SAUCE

Rich and elegant.

6 chicken breast halves, skin
and bone removed
½ cup butter
Salt and black pepper to taste
2 tablespoons sherry
2 teaspoons grated lemon peel
2 tablespoons lemon juice
1 cup whipping cream
Grated Parmesan cheese
Lemon slices for garnish

Sauté chicken in butter in large skillet, turning to lightly brown on both sides. Season with salt and black pepper and place in baking dish. Add sherry, lemon peel and juice to butter in skillet. Stir and cook for 3 to 4 minutes. Check seasoning. Stirring constantly, gradually add cream to sauce. Remove from heat and pour over chicken. Sprinkle Parmesan cheese on chicken. Bake at 350° for 20 to 30 minutes. Garnish with lemon slices.

Serves 6.

CHICKEN BREASTS PECAN

Using flat side of mallet, pound chicken breasts to flatten. Season flour with salt and black pepper. Lightly coat chicken with flour, dip into eggs and coat with pecans. Sauté chicken in 1 tablespoon butter in large skillet over medium heat, turning to brown on both sides. Place in baking dish. Bake at 375° for 15 minutes. While chicken is baking, deglaze skillet with wine. Add remaining 2 tablespoons butter and cook over low heat until thickened. Serve chicken with wine sauce.

Serves 4.

4   chicken breast halves, skin and bone removed
1   cup all-purpose flour
    Salt and black pepper to taste
2   eggs, beaten
¼   cup ground pecans
3   tablespoons butter, divided
¼   cup dry white wine

PISTACHIO CHICKEN WITH FRESH PEACHES

A delicious dish, worth the effort.

Using flat side of mallet, pound chicken breasts to ¼-inch thickness. Spread mustard on 1 side of chicken and sprinkle with ½ of pistachios. Layer ham over nuts. Roll up chicken, jelly roll style, and secure with wooden pick. Combine flour with remaining nuts and tarragon. Dip chicken bundles in egg, then in flour mixture. Melt butter in 13x9x2-inch baking dish. Arrange chicken bundles in baking dish. Bake at 375° for 20 minutes, add white wine and peach slices, and bake for additional 15 minutes.

Serves 4.

4   chicken breast halves, skin and bone removed
2   tablespoons Dijon mustard
¾   cup chopped pistachio nuts
¼   pound sliced prosciutto ham
2   tablespoons all-purpose flour
1   teaspoon chopped fresh tarragon
1   egg, beaten
¼   cup plus 2 tablespoons butter
¼   cup dry white wine
3   fresh peaches, peeled and sliced

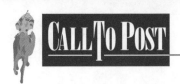
RASPBERRY CHICKEN EARL

6 chicken breast halves, skin and bone removed
¼ cup butter
½ cup minced onion
½ cup raspberry vinegar
½ cup chicken broth
½ cup half and half
2 tablespoons crushed tomatoes
½ cup frozen raspberries

Using flat side of mallet, lightly pound chicken breasts to flatten. Sauté chicken in butter in large skillet for about 3 minutes on each side. Remove chicken and set aside. Add onion to pan drippings and cook for 5 minutes. Stir in vinegar and cook, uncovered, until liquid is reduced to 2 tablespoons. Whisk broth, half and half and tomatoes into liquid. Simmer for 1 minute. Add chicken to sauce and simmer, basting often, for about 10 minutes or until chicken is done. Transfer chicken to platter. Add raspberries to sauce and simmer for 1 minute. Pour sauce over chicken.

Serves 6.

SPRING CHICKEN WITH FRESH VEGETABLE MEDLEY

Serve chicken and vegetables with rice or noodles.

4 chicken breast halves, skin and bone removed
   Salt and freshly ground black pepper
2 teaspoons olive oil
1¾ cups chicken broth
4 plum tomatoes, quartered
12 baby carrots
½ pound asparagus, trimmed and cut in 1½-inch pieces
1 yellow squash, cut in ¼-inch slices
1 leek, cleaned and cut in ¼-inch slices
1 cup fresh shelled peas

Season chicken with salt and black pepper. Sauté in oil in large skillet over medium-high heat, turning to brown on both sides. Add broth and tomatoes. Bring to a boil, reduce to medium-low heat and cook, covered, for about 20 minutes. Remove chicken and set aside. Add carrots to liquid in skillet and cook, covered, until nearly tender. Add asparagus, squash, leeks and peas. Cook until all vegetables are tender. Shred chicken into large bite-sized pieces and add to vegetables. Heat thoroughly.

Serves 4.

PHYLLO CHICKEN WITH FETA AND SPINACH

Add a green salad and what a meal!

Sauté onion in oil in large skillet over medium heat, stirring occasionally, until tender. Add spinach and cook, stirring frequently, until wilted. Remove skillet from heat and stir in feta cheese, wine, black pepper, egg and chicken. Place phyllo on flat surface. Trim to 16x12 inches. Working with 1 sheet at a time and keeping remaining sheets covered with plastic wrap and damp towel, brush sheet with melted butter and sprinkle with 1 tablespoon bread crumbs. Repeat process, stacking 5 sheets. Spread ½ of chicken mixture in 2-inch strip along short side of phyllo, leaving ½-inch margin. Roll up, jelly roll style, from chicken mixture edge. Repeat with remaining ingredients to form second roll. Place both, seam side down and 2 inches apart, on large baking sheet. Brush with butter. Using sharp knife, cut diagonally, halfway through phyllo layers, at 1 inch intervals. Bake at 375° for 15 to 20 minutes or until golden brown. Let stand for 10 minutes. Slice along cuts.

Serves 8.

1   medium onion, chopped
2   tablespoons olive oil
1   10-ounce bunch spinach, stemmed and chopped
¼   cup (1 ounce) crumbled feta cheese
2   tablespoons dry white wine
¼   teaspoon freshly ground black pepper
1   egg, lightly beaten
3   cups cubed cooked chicken
10 sheets frozen phyllo pastry, thawed
½   cup butter, melted
⅔   cup dry bread crumbs

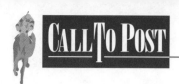

POLLO ROSSO

¼ cup chopped onion
2 tablespoons unsalted butter
2 tablespoons vegetable oil
1 clove garlic, minced
2 tablespoons sweet Hungarian paprika or to taste
1½ cups peeled, seeded and chopped ripe tomatoes or canned Italian style crushed tomatoes, with juice
1¼ cups fresh chicken broth or canned low-sodium broth
6 chicken breast halves, skin and bone removed
⅓ cup all-purpose flour
⅓ cup half and half or whipping cream
1 tablespoon sherry
Salt and freshly ground black pepper to taste
1 12-ounce package flat egg noodles
Minced fresh parsley for garnish

Sauté onion in butter and oil in heavy skillet over medium-high heat for 5 minutes or until softened. Add garlic and sauté for 1 to 2 minutes. Stir in paprika, tomatoes and broth. Cook, covered, for 10 minutes. Reduce heat, add chicken and simmer, covered, for 30 to 35 minutes or until chicken is tender but moist. Using slotted spoon, remove chicken and keep warm. Prepare noodles according to package directions, cooking until tender but firm. While noodles are cooking, blend flour and half and half or cream in small bowl. Add to simmering liquid in skillet and cook, stirring often, for about 10 minutes or until thickened. Stir in sherry. Season with salt and black pepper. Heat thoroughly but do not boil. Serve sauce over chicken and drained noodles.

Serves 6.

GRILLED CHICKEN WITH HOT PEPPER JELLY SAUCE

4 chicken breast halves
Salt and black pepper to taste
1 cup sweet hot pepper jelly
1 cup dry white wine
¼ cup chopped basil

Season chicken with salt and black pepper. Combine jelly, wine and basil in saucepan. Simmer over low heat to liquefy jelly. Use 1 cup sauce for marinating and basting chicken and remaining 1 cup for serving with chicken. Marinate chicken for 30 minutes. Grill over medium coals for about 8 minutes on each side or until done, basting frequently with sauce. Serve with additional sauce.

Serves 4.

WINE CHICKEN WITH RED BELL PEPPERS

Sauté bell peppers and garlic in butter and oil in heavy skillet over medium-high heat for about 10 minutes or until peppers are tender. Using slotted spoon, remove peppers and keep warm. Season chicken with salt and black pepper. Sprinkle flour on chicken. Sauté chicken, turning to lightly brown on both sides. Remove chicken from skillet. Return peppers to skillet and add broth and wine. Bring to a boil over high heat and cook, scraping to dislodge browned bits, for about 5 minutes or until thickened to sauce consistency. Add chicken and juices to sauce. Cook until chicken is done. Place chicken and sauce on platter and sprinkle with parsley.

Serves 4.

- 2 red bell peppers, thinly sliced
- 2 large cloves garlic, chopped
- 2 tablespoons butter
- 2 tablespoons olive oil
- 4 chicken breast halves, skin and bone removed
  Salt and black pepper to taste
  All-purpose flour
- 1 cup chicken broth
- ¼ cup dry white wine
- 2 tablespoons chopped fresh parsley

CHICKEN BREASTS WITH VERY BERRY MARINADE

Combine raspberries, vinegar, lemon juice, garlic, mint, black pepper and oil in blender or food processor. Blend thoroughly. Place chicken in shallow baking dish. Pour raspberry liquid over chicken. Marinate in refrigerator for 4 hours. Remove chicken from marinade. Grill over medium heat for about 4 minutes on each side or until done, basting frequently with marinade. Garnish with raspberries and mint.

Serves 8.

- ¾ cup puréed unsweetened raspberries
- 1 cup raspberry vinegar
- 2 tablespoons lemon juice
- 1 tablespoon minced garlic
- 2 tablespoons chopped fresh mint or 2 teaspoons dried
  Freshly ground black pepper to taste
- ⅓ cup olive oil
- 8 chicken breast halves, skin and bone removed
  Fresh raspberries for garnish
  Mint sprigs for garnish

159

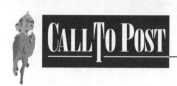
GRILLED BASIL CHICKEN

CHICKEN
¾ teaspoon coarsely ground
black pepper
4 chicken breast halves, skin
removed
⅓ cup olive oil
¼ cup chopped fresh basil

Press black pepper into meat sides of chicken breasts. Combine olive oil with basil, mixing well. Lightly brush on chicken. Grill chicken over medium coals for about 6 minutes on each side or until done, basting frequently with remaining melted butter. While chicken is cooking, prepare sauce. Serve chicken with sauce.

BASIL SAUCE
½ cup olive oil
2 tablespoons minced fresh
basil
1½ tablespoons grated Parmesan
cheese
½ teaspoon garlic powder
⅛ teaspoon salt
¼ teaspoon black pepper

Combine olive oil, basil, Parmesan cheese, garlic powder, salt and black pepper. Using electric mixer at low speed, mix until smooth.

Serves 4.

GRILLED CHICKEN AND VEGETABLES IN FOIL

4 chicken breast halves, skin
and bone removed
½ cup Italian salad dressing
4 new potatoes, sliced
1 green bell pepper, cut in
julienne strips
1 zucchini, cut in ¼-inch slices
2 medium onions, sliced
2 tomatoes, peeled and
quartered
Garlic salt to taste
Black pepper to taste

Marinate chicken in salad dressing for 3 hours or overnight in refrigerator. Place each chicken piece on 18x 14-inch aluminum foil sheet. Add potatoes, bell pepper, zucchini, onions and tomatoes to each chicken piece. Season with garlic salt and black pepper. Fold foil over ingredients and roll edges to seal, forming an envelope. Place on grill and cook for about 40 minutes or bake at 350° for 50 minutes or until chicken is thoroughly cooked, turning packets occasionally.

Serves 4.

GRILLED CITRUS CHICKEN

Combine oil, orange juice, lemon juice, rosemary, garlic, salt and white pepper in shallow baking dish. Add chicken, turning to coat well. Marinate, covered, for at least 6 hours or overnight in refrigerator, turning occasionally. Remove chicken from marinade. Grill over medium coals for about 5 minutes on each side until thoroughly cooked. Serve with garlic sauce.

Sauté garlic in oil in saucepan over medium-high heat until browned. Add broth, lemon juice, orange juice, salt and white pepper. Cook to reduce liquid by ½. Swirl in butter and allow to melt.

Serves 8.

CHICKEN
¼ cup olive oil
2 tablespoons lemon juice
2 tablespoons orange juice
1 tablespoon minced fresh rosemary
2 teaspoons minced garlic
2 teaspoons salt
1 teaspoon white pepper
8 chicken breast halves, skin and bone removed

GARLIC SAUCE
1 tablespoon minced garlic
2 teaspoons olive oil
¼ cup chicken broth
2 tablespoons fresh lemon juice
2 tablespoons orange juice
1 teaspoon salt
1 teaspoon white pepper
2 tablespoons unsalted butter, cut in bits

CHICKEN ENCHILADAS

Combine chicken, chilies, salsa, salt and garlic salt. Dip each tortilla in cream, fill with chicken mixture, roll to enclose and place in 2-quart casserole. Pour remaining cream over tortillas and sprinkle with cheese. Bake at 300° for 10 to 15 minutes or until warm and bubbly. Garnish with radishes and sour cream.

Serves 6.

2 cups cubed cooked chicken
2 4-ounce cans chopped green chilies, drained
½ cup salsa verde or medium-flavor red salsa
½ teaspoon salt
Garlic salt to taste
12 corn tortillas
2 cups whipping cream, warmed
2 cups (8 ounces) grated Mexican blend cheese
Radish slices for garnish
Sour cream for garnish

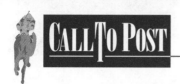

CHICKEN FAJITAS WITH LIME MARINADE

A fun south of the border dinner.

FAJITAS
- ½ cup vegetable oil
- 3 tablespoons white wine vinegar
- 2 tablespoons fresh lime juice
- 1 small onion, minced
- 1 clove garlic
- 1 teaspoon hot pepper sauce
- ½ teaspoon salt
- ¼ teaspoon freshly ground black pepper
- 8 chicken breast halves, skin and bone removed
- 16 flour tortillas, warmed
  Fresh tomato salsa
  Sour cream
  Shredded lettuce
  Black olives, sliced
  Freshly grated Cheddar cheese
  Guacamole (optional)

Combine oil, vinegar, lime juice, onion, garlic, hot pepper sauce, salt and black pepper in shallow baking dish. Add chicken and marinate for at least 1 hour at room temperature or overnight in refrigerator. While chicken is marinating, prepare salsa. Remove chicken, reserving marinade. Grill chicken over medium coals or broil, turning and basting with marinade several times, until chicken is opaque but moist. Cut in strips. To serve, spread tortillas with salsa and sour cream. Add chicken, lettuce, olives, Cheddar cheese and guacamole.

FRESH TOMATO SALSA
- 3 medium tomatoes, chopped
- 1 small onion, minced
- 1 jalapeño pepper, seeded and minced
- 2 tablespoons vegetable oil
- 1 tablespoon white wine vinegar
- ½ teaspoon salt
- ¼ cup fresh chopped cilantro

Combine tomatoes, onion, jalapeño pepper, oil, vinegar, salt and cilantro, mixing well.

Serves 8.

CHICKEN POT PIE

Easy...a family favorite!

Melt butter in saucepan over low heat. Blend in flour until smooth. Add broth and cook, stirring as it thickens to gravy consistency. Add milk, salt, black pepper, celery salt and garlic powder. Cook, stirring often, until smooth and bubbly. Add celery, onion and peas and carrots. Place chicken in 2-quart casserole. Pour sauce over chicken. Place pastry over sauce, crimping around edges to seal and cutting slit in pastry to vent steam. Place foil cuff around edges. Bake at 350° for 35 minutes, remove foil and bake until golden brown.

¼ cup butter
½ cup all-purpose flour
1 cup chicken broth
1 cup milk
½ teaspoon salt
⅛ teaspoon black pepper
⅛ teaspoon celery salt
¼ teaspoon garlic powder
¼ cup chopped celery
¼ cup chopped onion
1 10-ounce package frozen peas and carrots
2 cups cubed cooked chicken
1 unbaked 9-inch pastry shell

Serves 4.

CORNISH GAME HENS WITH SHERRY

Season all sides of hens with salt, black pepper and lemon juice. Place skin side up in baking pan. Dot with butter and add sherry. Bake at 325° for about 1 hour or until tender, basting occasionally with pan drippings; if liquid evaporates, add small amount of water. Remove from oven and brown hens under broiler. Remove hens from roasting pan. Blend flour with pan drippings, add mushrooms and juice and cook until thickened slightly. Pour sauce over hens. Serve with wild rice.

4 Cornish game hens, split
Salt and black pepper to taste
Juice of 1 lemon
½ cup butter
½ to ⅓ cup sherry
1 tablespoon all-purpose flour
½ pound mushrooms, sliced and sautéed

Serves 4.

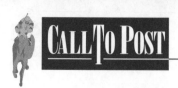
CHICKEN QUICHE WITH CHEDDAR PECAN CRUST

Perfect for a light luncheon.

PASTRY

1	cup all-purpose flour
1	cup (4 ounces) shredded sharp Cheddar cheese
¾	cup pecans, chopped
½	teaspoon salt
¼	teaspoon paprika
⅓	cup vegetable oil

Combine flour, Cheddar cheese, pecans, salt and paprika, mixing well. Stir in oil. Reserving ¼ of mixture, press remainder in bottom and along sides of 9-inch pie plate. Prick with fork tines. Bake at 350° for 10 minutes. Let stand until cool.

FILLING

3	eggs, beaten
½	cup chicken broth
1	cup sour cream
¼	cup mayonnaise
2	cups cubed cooked chicken
½	cup (2 ounces) shredded Cheddar cheese
2	tablespoons minced onion
½	teaspoon salt
¼	teaspoon dill weed
¼	cup pecan halves

Combine eggs, broth, sour cream and mayonnaise, blending well. Stir in chicken, Cheddar cheese, onion, salt and dill weed. Spoon mixture into baked crust. Sprinkle with reserved flour mixture and pecan halves. Bake at 350° for 45 minutes or until firm.

Serves 6.

SPLASH OF BOURBON MARINADE

¼	cup bourbon
¼	cup soy sauce
¼	cup Dijon mustard
¼	cup ketchup
¼	cup firmly-packed brown sugar
3	scallions, chopped
1	tablespoon minced rosemary

Combine bourbon, soy sauce, mustard and ketchup. Blend in brown sugar, scallions and rosemary. Marinate chicken in sauce for 1 to 2 hours.

Makes 1⅓ cups.

PINEAPPLE RUM MARINADE

Combine pineapple juice, rum, soy sauce, ginger root, garlic, brown sugar and black pepper, blending well. Pour marinade over chicken. Marinate, covered, in refrigerator for 4 to 8 hours, turning occasionally.

Makes 1¼ cups.

½ cup unsweetened pineapple juice
⅓ cup light rum
¼ cup soy sauce
1 tablespoon grated ginger root
2 cloves garlic, minced
1 tablespoon brown sugar
¼ teaspoon black pepper

DOVE AND OYSTER PIE

Place doves in large pot. Cover with water and add celery, onion, hot pepper sauce, salt, black pepper and Worcestershire sauce. Simmer until tender. Remove doves, reserving broth with celery and onion. After doves are cooled, remove meat and set aside. Combine flour with ¼ cup dove broth in saucepan and blend well over low heat. Add remaining broth with onion and celery. Cook, stirring frequently, until thickened. Remove from heat. Add oysters and mushrooms. Line 8x8x2-inch baking dish with 1 pastry shell. Bake at 350° for 5 minutes. Let stand until cool. Layer dove meat with broth mixture in partially baked pastry. Cover with remaining pastry shell. Bake at 350° until pastry is browned and pie is bubbly. Garnish with parsley and bacon.

Serves 6.

16 dove breasts
1 cup chopped celery
1 cup chopped onion
Several dashes hot pepper sauce
Salt and black pepper to taste
¼ cup plus 1 tablespoon Worcestershire sauce
All-purpose flour
1½ pints fresh select oysters
1½ cups sliced fresh mushrooms, sautéed
2 unbaked 9-inch pastry shells
¼ cup chopped parsley
12 slices bacon, cooked and crumbled

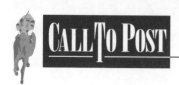

DOVE ON THE GRILL

12	doves
	Salt and black pepper to taste
	Jalapeño pepper juice
12	jalapeño peppers
12	slices fat bacon

Soak cleaned birds in salt water overnight to remove blood. Season birds liberally with salt and black pepper. Sprinkle with jalapeño pepper juice. Place 1 pepper in each bird between breast and bone or secure to breast with wooden pick. Wrap 1 slice bacon around breast and jalapeño pepper, securing with wooden pick. Grill until bacon is well done.

Serves 12.

QUAIL IN CHAFING DISH

8	quail
	Salt and black pepper to taste
½	cup butter
	Water
½	cup sherry
	Juice of 1½ lemons
¼	cup plus 1 tablespoon Worcestershire sauce
2½	tablespoons all-purpose flour
1	cup half and half

Season cleaned birds well with salt and black pepper. In Dutch oven, sauté birds breast side down with 1 teaspoon butter on each until lightly browned. Add water to keep birds from sticking to bottom of pot. Simmer, covered, for 1 hour. When nearly done, add sherry, lemon juice and Worcestershire sauce. Cook for about 20 minutes. Remove birds and set aside. Blend flour with half and half and stir into sauce. Simmer until thickened. Place birds and gravy in chafing dish. Ignite fuel to reheat. **Note:** Quail can be cooked early in afternoon and set aside to be reheated about 30 minutes before serving. Dove can be prepared in same way.

Serves 4.

QUAIL OR PHEASANT

Season birds with salt and black pepper. Lightly coat with flour. Sauté birds in butter in large skillet until lightly browned. Place birds in roasting pan or casserole. Remove excess fat from skillet. Add small amount of water to drippings and cook to dislodge browned bits. Stir in Worcestershire sauce and garlic. Pour sauce over birds and add lemon slices. Bake at 375° for 2 hours or until tender, basting occasionally with pan liquid. Add water to increase amount of gravy.

Serves 4.

8 quail or 2 3-pound pheasants
Salt and black pepper to taste
All-purpose flour
1 cup butter (not margarine)
1 teaspoon Worcestershire
sauce
Dash of garlic salt
2 or 3 slices lemon

PHEASANT RAGOUT

Cut pheasant meat into medium-sized pieces. Coat with flour and set aside. Sauté onion and garlic in butter in skillet for about 5 minutes or until vegetables are tender. Season with marjoram, salt and black pepper. Add pheasant pieces and cook, turning to brown on both sides. Place in casserole. Dissolve bouillon in boiling water. Pour bouillon over pheasant. Add wine and bay leaf. Bake, covered, at 300° for 2 hours or until pheasant is tender. Serve with wild rice, green vegetable and glazed butternut squash.

Serves 4.

Breasts and thighs of
2 pheasants, bones removed
3 tablespoons all-purpose flour
2 onions, sliced
2 cloves garlic, minced
½ cup butter
Pinch of marjoram
Dash of salt and black pepper
1 bouillon cube
1 cup boiling water
⅔ cup red wine
1 bay leaf

MEATS

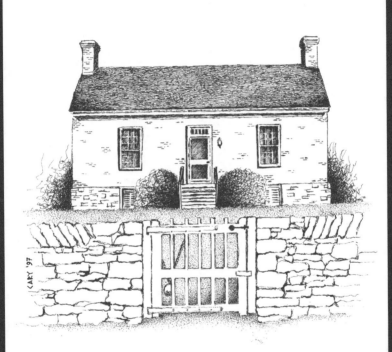

Founded and owned by Mr. and Mrs. William T. Young of Lexington, Overbrook Farm is located in Fayette County just south of the outskirts of Lexington and is the home of leading stallions, Storm Cat, Carson City, dual classic winner Tabasco Cat and Kentucky Derby winner Grindstone. One of the most successful racing stables of the nineties, Overbrook has bred more than sixty stakes winners.

Overbrook

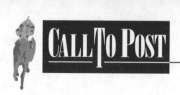

Meats

BEEF TENDERLOIN WITH WILD MUSHROOMS AND ASIAGO CHEESE

An elegant entrée.

Sauté mushrooms, green onion, garlic and parsley in butter until vegetables are softened. Cut tenderloin lengthwise, leaving ends connected to form large pocket. Sprinkle seasoned salt and black pepper inside pocket. Spoon mushroom mixture into pocket and sprinkle with Asiago cheese. Close tenderloin, securing with heavy cotton string at 2-inch intervals. Place in large shallow baking dish. Pour salad dressing over tenderloin. Chill, covered, for 8 hours, basting frequently with marinade. Remove from marinade and grill to rare doneness (140° on meat thermometer). Let stand for a few minutes before cutting in slices to serve.

2	pounds mixed wild mushrooms
2	cups chopped green onion
4	cloves garlic, minced
½	cup chopped fresh parsley
½	cup butter
1	6-pound beef tenderloin
¼	teaspoon seasoned salt
½	teaspoon freshly ground black pepper
4	ounces grated Asiago cheese
1	8-ounce bottle Italian salad dressing

Serves 12 to 16.

STUFFED FILET OF BEEF

Cut filets horizontally, leaving 1 side attached. Open each filet as if a book. Place 1 slice ham and Gruyère cheese on 1 side, then close and press edges together, securing with a wooden pick if necessary. Season filet with salt and black pepper. Coat thoroughly with flour, dip in egg and roll in bread crumbs. Sauté filet in butter in skillet for 5 minutes on each side or to desired degree of doneness.

4	beef filets (1½-inch thickness)
4	thin slices prosciutto ham
4	slices Gruyère cheese or other Swiss cheese
1	teaspoon salt
½	teaspoon freshly ground black pepper
¼	cup all-purpose flour
2	eggs
⅓	cup seasoned bread crumbs
5	tablespoons butter

Serves 4.

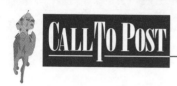

TENDERLOIN VERSAILLES

Well worth the effort...a delicious dish.

TENDERLOIN
- 4 cups low-sodium beef broth
- 1 carrot, chopped
- 1 onion, quartered
- 1 stalk celery, chopped
- 1 9-ounce jar chutney
- 1 teaspoon salt
- ½ teaspoon coarsely ground black pepper
- 1 tablespoon butter or margarine, softened
- 1 5 to 6-pound beef tenderloin, trimmed

  Wine reduction sauce
- 3 tablespoons butter
- ½ teaspoon chopped fresh thyme or ¼ teaspoon dried thyme

Combine broth, carrot, onion and celery in saucepan. Bring to a boil over medium heat, reduce heat and simmer for 40 minutes or until mixture is reduced to about 1½ cups. Strain into a bowl; reserve vegetables and set liquid aside. Using knife blade in food processor, process vegetables until smooth and set aside. Combine chutney, salt, black pepper and butter, stirring until smooth. Spread ½ of mixture evenly on all surfaces of tenderloin. Place tenderloin on rack in shallow roasting pan. Bake at 450° for 20 minutes. Remove from oven and spread remaining chutney mixture evenly over tenderloin. Bake for 10 to 20 additional minutes or until meat thermometer, inserted in thickest portion, registers 145° for rare or 160° for medium. While tenderloin is roasting, prepare wine reduction sauce. Remove tenderloin from pan and let stand 15 minutes before slicing. Remove rack from roasting pan. Add reserved broth to pan. Bring to a boil over medium heat, stirring to loosen browned bits. Pour into saucepan and add wine reduction sauce and vegetable mixture. Bring to a boil, reduce heat and simmer for 5 minutes, stirring frequently. Adding 1 tablespoon at a time, whisk in butter. Stir in thyme. Serve sauce with tenderloin.

Serves 12.

(Continued on next page)

(Tenderloin Versailles, continued)

Combine wine, shallots, bay leaf and thyme in small saucepan. Bring to a boil over medium heat, reduce heat and simmer for about 40 minutes or until liquid is reduced to 1 cup. Strain into measuring cup, pressing with back of spoon against sides of strainer to extract all liquid. Discard solids.

Makes 1 cup.

WINE REDUCTION SAUCE
1   750-milliliter bottle Cabernet Sauvignon (3 cups)
3   cloves shallots, minced
1   bay leaf
3   or 4 sprigs fresh thyme

MEDITERRANEAN STEW

Sauté beef and sausage in large skillet until browned. Drain excess fat. Cut sausage into slices and place with beef in Dutch oven. Add burgundy, water, tomato paste, salt, black pepper, garlic and paprika. Bring to a boil, reduce heat and simmer, covered, for 1½ to 2 hours or until meat is tender. Add ham, onion, bell pepper, parsley, beans and lemon peel. Simmer, covered, for about 20 minutes. Add cabbage and cook for about 15 minutes or until tender crisp. Chill stew overnight to develop flavors. Skim fat from surface and discard. Let stand until room temperature, then reheat for 15 to 20 minutes or until thoroughly hot.

Serves 6 to 8.

1   pound chuck steak, cut in 1½-inch cubes
1   pound sweet Italian sausage links
1½ cups burgundy
2   cups water
1   6-ounce can tomato paste
2   teaspoons salt
¾   teaspoon black pepper
3   cloves garlic, minced
2   teaspoons paprika
1   pound cooked ham, cubed
3   medium onions, coarsely chopped
1   red bell pepper, coarsely chopped
¼   cup chopped fresh parsley
2   16-ounce cans garbanzo beans, drained
1   teaspoon grated lemon peel
1   head cabbage, cut in wedges

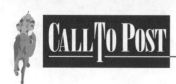

BLUEGRASS TOURNEDOS

½ cup sliced canned
mushrooms
2 tablespoons butter
1 tablespoon all-purpose flour
¼ cup red wine
½ cup mushroom liquid
½ teaspoon Worcestershire
sauce
¼ teaspoon salt
Dash of black pepper
4 small filet mignons
1 large ripe tomato

Sauté mushrooms in butter in small saucepan until tender. Stir in flour and cook over low heat for a few minutes or until lightly browned. Stir in wine, mushroom liquid, Worcestershire sauce, salt and black pepper. Cook until thickened. Season filets with salt and black pepper. Grill to desired degree of doneness. Cut tomato into 4 thick slices and grill just until warm. Arrange tomato slice on each filet and top with mushroom sauce.

Serves 4.

BEECH GROVE MEAT LOAF

1½ pounds lean ground beef or
venison
½ pound lean ground pork
1 cup minced onion
½ cup grated carrot
½ cup finely chopped celery
¼ cup finely chopped green
bell pepper
2 cloves garlic, minced
½ cup ketchup
3 eggs, beaten
½ cup half and half
1 teaspoon salt
1 teaspoon freshly ground
black pepper
¼ teaspoon cayenne pepper
½ teaspoon chili powder
¾ cup dry bread crumbs

Combine beef or venison, pork, onion, carrot, celery, green bell pepper and garlic. Add ketchup, eggs and half and half. Blend in salt, black pepper, cayenne pepper, chili powder and bread crumbs, mixing lightly but thoroughly. Shape into loaf and place in 9x5x3-inch loaf pan. Bake at 350° for 1 to 1¼ hours. Drain excess fat. Let loaf stand for about 10 minutes before cutting into slices.

Serves 6.

KENTUCKY BOURBON STEAK

Combine garlic, ginger root, bourbon, oil and soy sauce in food processor, blending thoroughly. Pour liquid over steak in shallow baking dish. Marinate, covered with plastic wrap, in refrigerator for 1 to 3 days. Prepare sauce and keep warm. Remove steak from marinade. Grill to desired degree of doneness. While steak is grilling, sauté onion. Cut steak in thin slices across the grain. Serve on onions with sauce.

Sauté mushrooms in butter for 2 minutes. Blend in flour and cook to form paste. Add ½ cup broth and blend thoroughly. Add remaining broth, Worcestershire sauce, salt and black pepper. Bring to a boil and cook for 5 minutes, stirring constantly. Reduce heat and simmer until thickened.

Serves 4.

STEAK AND MARINADE
5   cloves fresh garlic, chopped
1   1-inch piece ginger root, minced
¾   cup bourbon
½   cup olive oil
½   cup soy sauce
1   pound flank steak, cleaned and scored
1   medium onion, sliced and sautéed (optional)

SAUCE
1   cup sliced mushrooms
¼   cup clarified butter
¼   cup all-purpose flour
1½   to 2 cups beef broth
  Dash of Worcestershire sauce
1   ounce bourbon or to taste
  Salt and black pepper to taste

SPEEDY SAUERBRATEN

Sauté beef in butter in Dutch oven for 15 minutes, turning to brown on all sides. Add vinegar, water, onion, bay leaves, cloves, salt, black pepper and sugar. Simmer, covered, for 3 to 4 hours. Just before serving, add gingersnap crumbs to cooking liquid and simmer until thickened.

Serves 6 to 8.

3   pounds boneless chuck roast
2   tablespoons butter
1   cup vinegar
4   cups water
1   cup sliced onion
2   bay leaves
8   whole cloves
1½   teaspoons salt
  Dash of black pepper
2   tablespoons sugar
6   gingersnaps, crushed

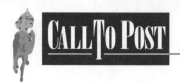

SANTA FE FLANK STEAK WITH FRUIT SALSA

Marinade and salsa work well with grilled pork tenderloin.

STEAK

1½ pounds flank steak
¼ cup fresh orange juice
2 tablespoons oil
2 tablespoons soy sauce
2 tablespoons chili sauce
2 tablespoons chili powder
1 teaspoon honey
1 teaspoon grated orange peel
½ teaspoon grated lemon peel
2 cloves garlic, minced
½ teaspoon salt
¼ teaspoon cayenne pepper
1 medium orange, peeled and thinly sliced
   Orange wedges for garnish
   Cilantro sprigs for garnish

Place steak in shallow baking dish. Combine orange juice, oil, soy sauce, chili sauce, chili powder, honey, orange peel, lemon peel, garlic, salt and cayenne pepper. Pour marinade over meat. Marinate, covered with plastic wrap, overnight in refrigerator. Prepare salsa. Bring steak to room temperature. Preheat grill. Drain marinade and discard. Grill steak for 4 to 6 minutes on each side or to desired degree of doneness. Cut steak diagonally into thin slices. Place on platter and surround with salsa. Garnish with orange wedges and cilantro sprigs.

FRESH FRUIT SALSA

1 cup diced pineapple
1 kiwi, peeled and sliced
1 cup chopped mango
¼ cup diced green bell pepper
½ cup diced red bell pepper
1½ tablespoons minced fresh cilantro
½ teaspoon crushed red pepper flakes
1 tablespoon plus 1 teaspoon sugar
2½ tablespoons white wine vinegar

Combine pineapple, kiwi, papaya, green bell pepper, red bell pepper, cilantro, red pepper flakes and sugar. Add vinegar and mix well. Chill, covered, overnight. Serve at room temperature.

Serves 3 or 4.

OLD FASHIONED MEAT LOAF

Complement this dish with garlic mashed potatoes and French style green beans.

Sauté onion and celery in butter in skillet for 3 to 5 minutes or until softened. Pour bread crumbs in bowl, pour milk over crumbs, stir and let stand until milk is absorbed. Add sautéed vegetables, beef, parsley, Worcestershire sauce, eggs, salt, black pepper, garlic powder and thyme to soaked crumbs, mixing well. Place bay leaves in bottom of 9x5x3-inch loaf pan. Shape mixture into loaf and place in pan. Bake at 350° for 1½ to 2 hours or until meat thermometer registers 160°. Let stand in pan, covered, for 5 minutes; drain excess fat and invert on serving platter. Remove bay leaves and cut in slices.

Serves 6 to 8.

1	medium onion, chopped
1	stalk celery, chopped
1	tablespoon unsalted butter
1½	cups crumbs from day-old French bread
½	cup milk
2	pounds ground sirloin
2	tablespoons chopped fresh parsley
1	teaspoon Worcestershire sauce
2	eggs, lightly beaten
1½	teaspoons salt
	Freshly ground black pepper
1	teaspoon garlic powder
¼	teaspoon dried thyme
2	bay leaves

ZUCCHINI BEEF BAKE

A wonderful way to enjoy vegetables.

Sauté beef and onion together in skillet until beef is browned, stirring to crumble. Drain excess fat. Combine beef mixture, zucchini, mushrooms, tomatoes, tomato sauce, salt, black pepper and paprika, mixing well. Spread mixture in 13x9x2-inch baking dish and top with bell pepper, mozzarella cheese and paprika. Bake at 350° for about 30 minutes or until bubbly.

Serves 6.

2	pounds ground chuck
1	onion, chopped
3	or 4 medium zucchini, sliced
1	pound mushrooms, sliced
1	pound Roma tomatoes, sliced
1	8-ounce can tomato sauce
	Salt and black pepper to taste
1	tablespoon chopped fresh basil
1	green bell pepper, chopped
1	cup (4 ounces) shredded mozzarella cheese
	Paprika

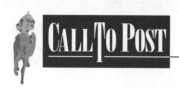

VEAL CHOPS WITH FONTINA CHEESE, SUN-DRIED TOMATOES AND VERMOUTH

½ cup pine nuts
7 tablespoons unsalted butter
6 thinly cut boneless veal loin
    chops
    Salt and freshly ground black
    pepper
1 cup dry vermouth
12 pieces oil-packed sun-dried
    tomatoes, drained and finely
    chopped
1 cup grated fontina cheese
6 lemon wedges
    Fresh watercress or fresh
    parsley sprigs for garnish

Sauté pine nuts in 1 tablespoon butter in small skillet over low heat, stirring constantly, until nuts are very light brown. Using smooth side of mallet, pound chops until very thin. Sauté chops in remaining ¼ cup plus 2 table-spoons butter in heavy skillet, browning quickly on both sides and turning only once. Season with salt and black pepper. Add vermouth and tomatoes. Simmer for about 12 minutes or until liquid is reduced to small amount. Spoon sauce over chops and sprinkle with pine nuts and fontina cheese. Broil until cheese is melted. Serve with lemon wedges and garnish with watercress or parsley.

Serves 6.

GRILLED LAMB BURGERS

1¾ pounds lean ground lamb
½ cup chopped fresh mint
3 large cloves garlic, finely
    minced
    Grated zest of 1 lemon
¼ cup fresh lemon juice
1 teaspoon salt
    Freshly ground black pepper
    to taste
    Fresh mint sprigs for garnish
    Lemon wedges for garnish

Blot lamb with paper towels to dry. Combine lamb, mint, garlic and lemon zest, mixing with hands. Blend in lemon juice; mixture will be moist but will hold together. Season with salt and black pepper. Shape lamb into 10 thin patties. Chill, covered, until ready to grill. Grill patties 4 to 6 inches above hot coals or broil 4 to 5 inches below heat source, turning once, for 5 to 8 minutes or until browned on outside and slightly pink on inside. Garnish servings with mint sprigs and lemon wedges.

Serves 5.

VEAL SCALLOPINE DIJON

Place veal between wax paper sheets and pound with smooth side of mallet. Season lightly with salt and black pepper and coat lightly with flour. Sauté cutlets in butter, turning to lightly brown on each side. Transfer veal to serving plate. Drain excess fat from pan and deglaze with wine. Cook to reduce wine liquid. Add cream and cook to reduce liquid. Stir in mustard, basil and tarragon. Serve sauce with veal. **Note:** To clarify butter, simmer to melt. Skim foamy material that accumulates on surface. Carefully separate clarified butter from milk solids that settle to bottom of pan.

Serves 4.

1½ to 2 pounds veal cutlets
Salt and black pepper to taste
All-purpose flour
1¾ cups clarified butter
½ cup dry white wine
3 cups whipping cream
2 tablespoons Dijon mustard
1 tablespoon dried basil
1 tablespoon dried tarragon

HERB ROASTED LEG OF LAMB

Combine garlic, salt and oil. Spread mixture on surface of lamb. Sprinkle marjoram, rosemary, thyme and flour on lamb. Place lamb in roasting pan. Combine wine and water. Pour over lamb. Bake at 325° for 2½ hours, basting frequently with pan juices.

Serves 8 to 10.

2 tablespoons crushed and minced garlic
1 teaspoon salt
2 tablespoons vegetable oil
1 6-pound leg of lamb
1 tablespoon minced fresh marjoram or 1 teaspoon dried marjoram
1 tablespoon minced fresh rosemary or 1 teaspoon dried rosemary
1 tablespoon minced fresh thyme or 1 teaspoon dried thyme
2 tablespoons all-purpose flour
1 cup dry white wine
1 cup water

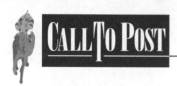
VEAL CUTLETS WITH LIME

2 tablespoons minced fresh parsley
1½ teaspoons lime zest, divided
½ teaspoon minced garlic
¼ cup all-purpose flour
1 teaspoon tarragon
Salt and black pepper to taste
8 veal cutlets (1½ inches thick)
3 tablespoons unsalted butter
1½ tablespoons olive oil
¾ cup dry white wine
1 tablespoon fresh lime juice
1 lime, thinly sliced, for garnish

Combine parsley, ½ teaspoon lime zest and garlic. Set aside. On wax paper sheet, mix flour, remaining 1 teaspoon lime zest, tarragon, salt and black pepper. Using smooth side of mallet, pound cutlets to ⅛-inch thickness. Lightly coat cutlets in seasoned flour, shaking to remove excess, and place cutlets on separate wax paper sheet. Heat butter and oil together in large heavy skillet over moderately high heat until sizzling. Reduce heat to moderate. Sauté cutlets, 2 at a time, for about 30 seconds on each side or until lightly browned. Transfer cutlets to heatproof dish and keep warm at 200° in oven. Pour wine into skillet and cook, scraping to dislodge any brown bits, for about 2 minutes or until liquid is reduced to ½ cup. Stir in parsley mixture and lime juice. Using tongs, dip each cutlet in sauce and arrange on individual dinner plates or platter. Spoon remaining sauce over cutlets and garnish with lime slices.

Serves 8.

THAI MARINATED PORK LOIN

1 cup crunchy peanut butter
½ cup prepared chili sauce
¼ cup lime juice
½ cup soy sauce
⅓ cup chopped fresh cilantro
¼ cup firmly-packed brown sugar
8 green onions, chopped
3 tablespoons chopped garlic
1 teaspoon salt
½ teaspoon black pepper
4 pork tenderloins

Combine peanut butter, chili sauce, lime juice, soy sauce, cilantro, brown sugar, green onion, garlic, salt and black pepper. Trim membranes from pork tenderloin. Thoroughly coat pork with marinade. Chill, covered, for at least 3 hours or overnight if possible. Drain marinade. Grill pork for about 15 to 20 minutes or until a meat thermometer registers 160°.

Serves 8.

ASHLAND LEG OF LAMB

Marinade is also great on beef.

Trim excess fat and membranes from lamb. Place in glass or plastic container. Combine garlic, shallots, ginger root, red pepper flakes, black pepper, lime juice and ¼ cup oil, blending well. Combine soy sauce and honey in small saucepan and heat until blended. Add warm liquid to lime juice mixture. Pour marinade over lamb, turning to coat all sides. Store, covered with plastic wrap, overnight in refrigerator. Bring to room temperature before roasting. Heat remaining ¼ cup oil in large heavy roasting pan on stove top. Place lamb, smooth side down, in pan and sear until well browned; turn to brown other side. Bake at 425° for 20 to 25 minutes for medium to rare doneness. Place on carving board and let stand 5 minutes before slicing.

Serves 8 to 10.

1   5½ to 6-pound leg of lamb, boned and butterflied
3   large cloves garlic, minced
3   shallots, finely chopped
¼   cup finely chopped ginger root
¼   teaspoon crushed red pepper flakes
1   tablespoon coarsely ground black pepper
¼   cup lime juice
½   cup vegetable oil, divided
¼   cup soy sauce
1   tablespoon honey

HONEY MUSTARD PORK KABOBS

Combine mustard, honey, garlic, lemon juice, jalapeño pepper, salt and black pepper, whisking to blend. Reserve 1 tablespoon marinade for basting. Add remaining marinade to pork in bowl. Toss pork pieces to coat and let stand for 1 hour. Thread pork on 4 10-inch metal skewers. Grill on oiled rack 5 to 6 inches above glowing coals for 5 minutes. Turn kabobs, baste with reserved marinade, and continue turning and basting for 10 to 15 minutes or until pork is cooked and registers 160° on meat thermometer.

Serves 2.

¼   cup Dijon mustard
2   tablespoons honey
2   large cloves garlic, minced
2   tablespoons fresh lemon juice
2   fresh jalapeño peppers, seeded and minced
    Salt and black pepper to taste
2   pork tenderloins, trimmed and cut crosswise in 1½-inch slices

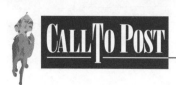
GARLIC HERBED LAMB SHANKS

6 cloves garlic, minced
2 teaspoons salt, divided
½ teaspoon freshly ground
   black pepper
4 lamb shanks
2 tablespoons all-purpose flour
2 tablespoons olive oil
1½ cups sliced onion
3 tablespoons chopped fresh
   mint
1 tablespoon chopped fresh
   parsley
2 tablespoons chopped fresh
   rosemary
1 tablespoon fresh thyme
   leaves
1 cup white wine
3 cups veal or chicken broth

Combine 1 teaspoon garlic, 1 teaspoon salt and black pepper. Rub mixture on all surfaces of lamb shanks. Coat shanks with flour. Sauté shanks in oil in Dutch oven or large ovenproof skillet over medium heat, turning to brown on all sides. Remove shanks from pan and set aside. Sauté onion and remaining 5 teaspoons garlic in oil for 3 to 5 minutes or until softened. Add mint, parsley, rosemary and thyme. Cook for 5 minutes. Pour wine into pan and cook over high heat until liquid is reduced by ½. Stir in broth, season with remaining 1 teaspoon salt and ¼ teaspoon black pepper. Bring to a simmer. Place shanks in pan. Bake, covered, at 325° for 2 hours or until meat is fork tender. Remove cover and increase oven temperature to 500°. Brown shanks in oven for 20 minutes, basting thoroughly with pan liquid. Remove shanks and set aside. Cook sauce over high heat to reduce by ½. Serve shanks whole with gravy ladled over them or remove meat, return to pan and serve as stew over rice or potatoes.

Serves 4 to 6.

GRILLED MARINATED PORK TENDERLOIN

Marinade can be prepared 2 days in advance and stored, covered, in refrigerator. Reheat before serving.

Combine garlic, soy sauce, ginger root, mustard, lime juice, oil, salt, black pepper and cayenne pepper in blender or food processor, blending well. Pour marinade into large sealable plastic bag and add tenderloins. Pressing out excess air, seal bag and place in shallow baking dish. Marinate in refrigerator, turning occasionally, for 3 to 6 hours. Let pork stand at room temperature about 30 minutes before grilling. Remove from marinade, allowing excess to drain. Grill on oiled rack 5 to 6 inches above the heat for 15 to 20 minutes or until meat thermometer registers 160°. Place pork on cutting board and let stand for 5 minutes before slicing. Serve with jalapeño onion chutney.

MARINADE

- 6 large cloves garlic, chopped
- 2 tablespoons soy sauce
- 2 tablespoons grated ginger root
- 2 teaspoons Dijon mustard
- ⅓ cup fresh lime juice
- ½ cup olive oil
  Salt and black pepper to taste
  Cayenne pepper to taste
- 4 pork tenderloins

Sauté onion in oil, seasoned with salt and black pepper, in large heavy skillet over medium heat until onion is softened. Add jalapeños and cook for 1 minute, stirring frequently. Add honey and stir-cook for 1 minute. Pour in vinegar and simmer, stirring, until nearly all liquid is evaporated. Add water and simmer, stirring, for about 10 minutes or until slightly thickened and onions are very tender. Season with salt and black pepper.

Serves 8 to 10.

JALAPEÑO ONION CHUTNEY

- 1¼ pounds red or yellow onions, finely chopped
- 3 tablespoons olive oil
  Salt and black pepper to taste
- 2 jalapeño peppers, seeded and minced
- 2 tablespoons honey
- 3 to 4 tablespoons red wine vinegar
- ¼ cup water

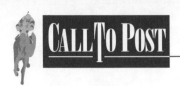

GRILLED PORK TENDERLOIN WITH PORT AND DRIED CHERRIES

1	cup olive oil
¼	cup dry vermouth
3	tablespoons chopped fresh thyme or 2 teaspoons dried thyme, crumbled
1	teaspoon salt
2	teaspoons black pepper
3	cloves garlic, minced
6	pork tenderloins (about 3½ pounds), well trimmed
1	750-milliliter bottle Cabernet Sauvignon (3 cups)
1	tablespoon minced shallot
2	cups whipping cream
½	cup dried cherries

Combine oil, vermouth, thyme, salt, black pepper and garlic in large shallow baking dish, whisking to blend. Add pork. Chill, covered, overnight, turning occasionally. Pour wine into saucepan. Bring to a boil and cook to reduce to 1 cup. Add shallots and cream. Boil to reduce liquid by ½. Stir in cherries and simmer for 3 to 5 minutes or until cherries are softened. Season sauce with salt and black pepper. Cover and keep warm. Drain marinade from pork. Grill pork on oiled rack about 4 inches above glowing coals for 5 to 6 minutes on each side or until meat thermometer registers 160°. Place on carving board and let stand for 10 minutes before diagonally slicing. Serve with sauce.

Serves 8 to 10.

VENISON WITH COLA MARINADE

1	3- to 4-pound venison roast
2	cloves garlic, minced
2	tablespoons vegetable oil
1	cup cola-flavored soft drink
1¼	teaspoons salt
¼	teaspoon black pepper
¼	teaspoon dry mustard
1	tablespoon white vinegar
2	tablespoons soy sauce
1	tablespoon ketchup

Place roast in shallow baking dish and set aside. Sauté garlic in oil in small skillet. Add cola, salt, black pepper, mustard, vinegar, soy sauce and ketchup, mixing well. Pour marinade over roast. Marinate, covered, for 8 hours in refrigerator, turning occasionally. Remove roast and reserve marinade. Place roast on large rectangle of heavy-duty aluminum foil. Bring edges of foil up around roast, leaving top open. Place in baking pan. Pour marinade over roast. Bake at 325° for 2½ hours or until meat thermometer registers 170°, basting with marinade at 45 minute intervals.

Serves 10 to 12.

CAKES & PIES

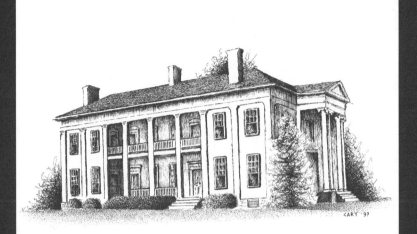

Six generations of Walden ancestors, dating back to 1810, have occupied the fertile Woodford County land on Weisenberger Mill Road near Midway, now called Vinery, and owned by Mr. and Mrs. Benjamin Parrish Walden, Jr.

Vinery's roster of 33 stallions, the largest in America, includes leading sires Red Ransom and Farma Way, plus Horse-of-the-Year Black Tie Affair and Kentucky Derby winner Strike the Gold.

The residence at Vinery, built in 1847, is designated a National Historic Landmark. It became the official "Residence" in 1994, when the former brick home to generations of Waldens, circa 1810, was converted into the Vinery office quarters.

Vinery

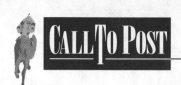

Cakes & Pies

E'S FRESH APPLE CAKE

Wonderful for breakfast, lunch or dinner!

Combine sugar, oil and eggs, mixing well. Mix flour, baking soda, salt, cinnamon and cloves or ginger together. Add to egg mixture. Fold in apples and pecans or raisins. Pour batter into greased and floured 10-inch tube pan or fluted tube pan. Bake at 325° for 1 hour. Cool in pan for 10 minutes, then invert on wire rack. Prepare glaze and pour over cake.

Combine brown sugar, milk and butter in saucepan. Bring to a boil and cook for 3 minutes.

Serves 12.

CAKE
- 2 cups sugar
- 1¼ cups vegetable oil
- 3 eggs
- 3 cups all-purpose flour
- 1 teaspoon baking soda
- 1 teaspoon salt
- 2 teaspoons cinnamon
  Pinch of ground cloves or ginger
- 3 cups peeled and chopped tart cooking apples
- 1 cup chopped pecans or raisins (optional)

GLAZE
- 1 cup firmly-packed brown sugar
- ¼ cup evaporated milk
- ½ cup butter, softened

PEAR CAKE

Cream butter and ¾ cup sugar together until light and fluffy. Add eggs and mix well. Combine flour, baking powder and salt. Add dry ingredients and vanilla to creamed mixture, mixing thoroughly. Spread batter in 9-inch springform pan. Distribute pears evenly on batter, dot with butter and sprinkle with remaining ¼ cup sugar. Bake at 350° for 1 hour. Cool in pan for 10 minutes, then invert on wire rack to cool completely. Cake is better if not refrigerated.

Serves 8.

- ½ cup butter, softened
- 1 cup sugar, divided
- 2 eggs
- 1 cup all-purpose flour
- ½ teaspoon baking powder
- ½ teaspoon salt
- ½ teaspoon vanilla
- 2 pounds ripe pears, peeled, cored and sliced
- 2 tablespoons butter, firm
- ¼ cup sugar

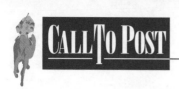

LIGHT BLUEBERRY POUND CAKE

Ideal to serve with brunch or light dinner.

CAKE
- 1 cup low-fat margarine, softened
- 2 cups sugar
- ½ cup egg substitute (2 egg equivalent)
- 1 teaspoon vanilla
- 2 cups all-purpose flour
- 1 teaspoon baking powder
- 1 cup low-fat sour cream
  Cinnamon sugar
- 2 cups fresh blueberries

Cream margarine and sugar together until light and fluffy. Add egg and vanilla and mix thoroughly. Sift flour and baking powder together. Alternately add dry ingredients and sour cream to creamed mixture. Spread ½ of batter in 10-inch fluted tube pan or angel food cake pan prepared with vegetable cooking spray. Distribute blueberries evenly on batter, pressing lightly, and sprinkle with cinnamon sugar. Spoon remaining batter on blueberries and sprinkle with cinnamon sugar. Bake at 350° for 50 to 60 minutes. Cool in pan for 10 minutes, then invert on wire rack to complete cooling. Drizzle glaze over cooled cake.

GLAZE
- ½ cup powdered sugar, sifted
- 2 tablespoons lemon juice

Blend sugar and lemon juice together until smooth.

Serves 12 to 16.

WINNING CARROT CAKE

Combine eggs and sugar, beating until sugar is dissolved. Blend in oil. Sift flour, baking powder, baking soda, salt and cinnamon together. Add dry ingredients, carrots, pineapple and nuts to egg mixture, mixing well. Spread batter in 3 greased and floured 9-inch round baking pans. Bake at 350° for 35 to 40 minutes. Cool in pans for 10 minutes, then invert on wire racks to cool completely. Spread frosting between cake layers, stack and spread on sides and tops of assembled cake.

Cream butter or margarine, cream cheese and vanilla together until smooth. Gradually add sugar and beat thoroughly.

Serves 12 to 16.

CAKE
- 4 eggs, beaten
- 2 cups sugar
- 1½ cups vegetable oil
- 2 cups all-purpose flour
- 2 teaspoons baking powder
- 1½ teaspoons baking soda
- 1 teaspoon salt
- 2 teaspoons cinnamon
- 2 cups grated carrots
- 1 8½-ounce can crushed pineapple, drained
- ½ cup chopped nuts

CREAM CHEESE FROSTING
- 1 cup butter or margarine, softened
- 2 8-ounce packages cream cheese, softened
- 2 teaspoons vanilla
- 4 cups powdered sugar, sifted

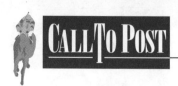

HUMMINGBIRD CAKE

CAKE
- 3 cups all-purpose flour
- 1 teaspoon baking soda
- 1 teaspoon salt
- 1 teaspoon cinnamon
- 3 eggs
- 2 cups sugar
- 1½ cups vegetable oil
- 1 8½-ounce can crushed pineapple
- 1 cup chopped walnuts
- 3 ripe bananas, mashed

CREAM CHEESE FROSTING
- 1 cup unsalted butter, softened
- 1 8-ounce package cream cheese, softened
- 1 teaspoon vanilla
- 1 16-ounce package powdered sugar, sifted

Combine flour, baking soda, salt and cinnamon. In order listed and mixing well with wooden spoon after each ingredient, add eggs, sugar, oil, pineapple, walnuts and bananas; do not use electric mixer. Spread batter in 3 9-inch round baking pans prepared with vegetable cooking spray. Bake at 350° for 30 minutes or until cake separates slightly from side of pan. Cool in pans for 10 minutes, then invert on wire racks to cool completely. Spread frosting between cake layers, stack and spread on sides and tops of assembled cake.

Cream butter, cream cheese and vanilla together until smooth. Gradually add sugar and beat thoroughly.

Serves 12 to 16.

SOUR CREAM POUND CAKE

Gorgeous cake—very light...this won't last long.

- 1 cup butter, softened
- 3 cups sugar
- 6 eggs, separated
- 3 cups sifted cake flour
- ¼ teaspoon baking soda
- 1 cup sour cream
- 1 teaspoon vanilla or almond extract
  Powdered sugar, sifted (optional)

Cream butter, gradually adding sugar and beating until smooth. Add egg yolks, 1 at a time, beating after each addition. Sift flour and baking soda together. Alternately add dry ingredients and sour cream to creamed mixture. Beat egg whites until stiff. Fold into batter. Stir in vanilla or almond extract. Spread batter in greased and floured 10-inch tube pan or fluted tube pan. Bake at 300° for 1½ hours or until wooden pick inserted in center comes out clean. Cool in pan for 10 minutes, then invert on wire rack to cool completely. Sprinkle powdered sugar over cake.

LOLA MURRAY'S CREAM CHEESE POUND CAKE

Outstanding!

Cream butter and cream cheese together until smooth. Add sugar and beat until light and fluffy. Add eggs, 1 at a time, beating 1 minute after each addition. Combine flour and baking powder. Gradually blend dry ingredients into egg mixture. Stir in vanilla and lemon extract. Spread batter in greased and floured 10-inch tube. Place in cold oven and set oven temperature at 300°. Bake, covered with aluminum foil, for 30 minutes; remove foil and bake for additional 50 to 60 minutes.

CAKE

1½   cups butter, softened
1   8-ounce package cream cheese softened
3   cups sugar
6   eggs
3   cups cake flour, sifted
¼   teaspoon baking powder
1½   teaspoons vanilla
1   teaspoon lemon extract

Beat butter, vanilla and milk together until smooth. Gradually add sugar and beat thoroughly.

Serves 8 to 10.

FROSTING

½   cup butter, softened
1   teaspoon vanilla
1   to 2 tablespoons milk
1   16-ounce package powdered sugar, sifted

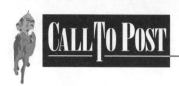

JAM CAKE

A must for the holidays!

CAKE
- 1 cup raisins
- 2 cups hot water
- 1 cup butter, softened
- 2 cups sugar
- 5 eggs
- 1 teaspoon baking soda
- 1 cup buttermilk
- 2 teaspoons vanilla or bourbon
- 3 cups all-purpose flour
- ¼ teaspoon salt
- 1½ teaspoons allspice
- ½ teaspoon cinnamon
- 1½ teaspoons cloves
- 1 cup blackberry jam
- 1½ cups chopped nuts, divided

Combine raisins and hot water and set aside to soak. Cream butter and sugar together until light and fluffy. Add eggs, 1 at a time, beating well after each addition. Dissolve soda in buttermilk. Blend in vanilla and add liquid to egg mixture. Mix in dry ingredients. Add jam and 1 cup nuts. Drain raisins, pressing to remove all excess moisture. Chop quickly in food processor. Add raisins to batter. Spread batter in 3 greased and floured 9-inch round cake pans. Bake at 325° for 40 minutes. Cool in pan for 10 minutes, then invert on wire rack to complete cooling. Spread frosting between cake layers, stack and spread on sides and tops of assembled cake. Sprinkle with remaining ½ cup nuts.

FROSTING
- ½ cup butter
- 1 cup firmly-packed brown sugar
- ½ teaspoon salt
- ¼ cup cream
- 1½ cups powdered sugar, sifted

Melt butter in saucepan over low heat. Stir in brown sugar and salt. Stirring constantly, bring mixture to a boil. Remove from heat, stir in cream, return to heat, bring to a boil and remove from heat. Using electric mixer, beat in powdered sugar until spreading consistency. If frosting thickens while being spread on cake, thin with small amount of cream. Sprinkle with remaining ½ cup nuts.

Serves 12.

MRS. MOPPETT'S WHITE CHOCOLATE CAKE WITH WHITE CHOCOLATE FROSTING

Combine white chocolate and water in double boiler, reduce heat until it melts, let cool. Cream butter and sugar well. Add egg yolks 1 at a time beating 1 minute after each addition. Add chocolate mixture and vanilla. Combine flour, soda, salt and add to cream mixture–alternately with buttermilk, ending with the flour mixture. Beat egg whites at room temperature until soft peaks form, fold whites into batter. Pour into 3 greased and floured 9-inch cake pans. Bake at 350° for 30 minutes. Cool in pan 10 minutes and remove.

4	ounces white chocolate broken into bits
½	cup water
1	cup butter, softened
2	cups sugar
4	eggs, separated
1	teaspoon vanilla
2½	cups sifted cake flour
1	teaspoon baking soda
½	teaspoon salt
1	cup buttermilk

Combine first 4 ingredients in double broiler. Reduce to low and cook until thick. Add in white chocolate until melted. Frost cooled cake.

WHITE CHOCOLATE FROSTING

3	egg yolks beaten
1	cup sweetened condensed milk
1	cup sugar
½	cup butter, melted
4	ounces white chocolate, grated

SPRINGS FAMOUS PECAN PIE

Cream butter and sugar together until smooth. Add salt, eggs, syrup and pecans. Mix thoroughly. Spread filling in pastry shell. Bake at 300° for 1 hour or until knife tip inserted 1 inch from edge comes out clean.

Serves 6 to 8.

2	tablespoons butter, softened
1	cup sugar
¼	teaspoon salt
2	eggs, well beaten
1	cup light corn syrup
1	cup chopped pecans
1	unbaked 9-inch pastry shell

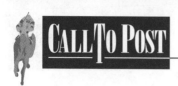

CHOCOLATE POUND CAKE

1 cup butter
½ cup Crisco
3 cups sugar
5 eggs

Cream first 3 ingredients. Add eggs 1 at a time, beating 1 minute each.

SIFT TOGETHER
3 cups flour
½ cup cocoa
¼ teaspoon salt
½ teaspoon baking powder

Add alternately to #1 with 1¼ cups milk, then add 1 teaspoon vanilla. Bake in a greased and floured bundt or tube pan for 1 hour and 20 minutes. Let cool in pan 10 minutes then remove from pan and cool completely before icing.

ICING
3 tablespoons water
4 tablespoons sugar

Boil water with sugar and remove from heat.

CREAM
⅔ cup Crisco
1 box powdered sugar
1 egg
4 tablespoons cocoa
1 teaspoon vanilla

In a slow drip, add water mixture to creamed mixture.

Serves 20.

EASY CHOCOLATE PIE

4 eggs, lightly beaten
2 cups sugar
1 cup all-purpose flour
2 teaspoons vanilla
1 cup butter
1 12-ounce package semisweet chocolate chips
2 unbaked 9-inch pastry shells

Using electric mixer, beat eggs and sugar together. Add flour and vanilla, mixing well. Melt butter and chocolate together in saucepan over low heat. Blend chocolate mixture into batter. Pour filling into pastry shells. Bake at 350° for 30 minutes.

Serves 12.

THE COOKSHOP RUM CAKE

Cream butter and sugars until smooth. Add rum, vanilla extract and milk, and blend well, scraping the bowl often. Add eggs, one at a time, beating well after each egg. Combine flour, salt and baking soda and add to batter, beating until smooth. Spread batter into a greased and floured bundt pan. Bake at 325° for 1 hour and 15 minutes. Remove cake from oven but leave it in the pan.

Combine orange juice and sugar over low heat until sugar has dissolved. Remove from heat and add rum, stirring to combine. Pour warm glaze over the cake and let soak in the pan for 15 minutes. Turn cake out of pan to cool.

1	cup unsalted butter, softened
½	cup sugar
1½	cups dark brown sugar
½	cup dark rum
1	tablespoon pure vanilla extract
¾	cup milk
5	eggs
3	cups all-purpose flour
¾	teaspoon salt
½	teaspoon baking soda

GLAZE

¼	cup orange juice
½	cup sugar
½	cup dark rum

TOASTED COCONUT PIE

Combine eggs, sugar, butter or margarine, lemon juice and vanilla, mixing thoroughly. Stir in coconut. Pour filling into pastry shell. Bake at 350° for 40 to 45 minutes or until firm. Cool slightly before serving. Serve with dollops of whipped cream or topping and garnish with toasted coconut.

Serves 6 to 8.

3	eggs, beaten
1½	cups sugar
½	cup butter or margarine, melted
1	tablespoon plus 1 teaspoon lemon juice
1	teaspoon vanilla
1⅓	cups flaked coconut
1	unbaked 9-inch pastry shell
1	cup coconut, toasted

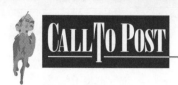

LEMON MERINGUE PIE

PIE
- 1 refrigerated 9-inch pastry crust, at room temperature
- 1 teaspoon all-purpose flour
- 1¼ cups sugar
- 1½ cups water
- ¼ cup plus 1 tablespoon cornstarch
- 5 egg yolks
- 1 tablespoon grated lemon peel
- Pinch of salt
- ½ cup fresh lemon juice
- 2 tablespoons unsalted butter, softened

Unfold pastry, pressing and moistening to smooth fold lines. Lightly sprinkle flour on crust and place, floured side down, in 9-inch pie plate. Crimp edges and prick with fork tines on bottom and sides. Bake on center rack at 450° for 12 minutes or until golden. Cool on wire rack. Combine sugar, water, cornstarch, egg yolks, lemon peel and salt together in saucepan, whisking to blend. Bring to a boil, whisking frequently, and cook for 2 minutes or until thickened. Remove from heat. Add lemon juice and butter and whisk until smooth. Let stand for about 1 hour or until cool, stirring occasionally.

MERINGUE
- ⅓ cup sugar
- 1 tablespoon cornstarch
- 5 egg whites
- ½ teaspoon cream of tartar

Combine sugar and cornstarch. Beat egg whites until foamy, add cream of tartar and beat until stiff peaks form. Add dry ingredients, 1 tablespoon at a time, to egg whites, beating after each addition until stiff peaks form. Pour cooled filling into pastry shell. Spread meringue over filling, sealing completely to pastry edge. Use spoon to swirl meringue. Bake at 350° for 12 minutes or until meringue peaks are lightly browned. Cool pie on rack, then store in refrigerator for about 1½ hours or until cold.

Serves 6 to 8.

COOKIES & CANDIES

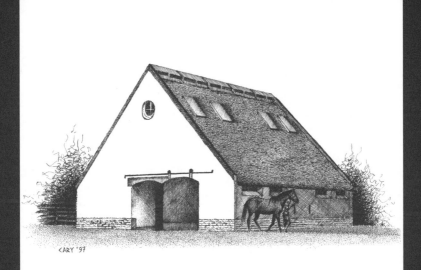

CARY '97

Gainesway is located at 3750 Paris Pike on some of the most historic Thoroughbred land in the Bluegrass region. The Gainesway Stallion Complex was voted one of the world's best architectural projects in 1984 by the American Institute of Architects. Owned by Graham J. Beck, Gainesway currently stands 17 stallions and is home to Broad Brush and Cozzene, America's Leading Thoroughbred sires of 1994 and 1996, respectively. Surrounding the stallion complex are over 1,000 acres for the boarding of clients' broodmares. Gainesway is a full-service operation which includes sales prep, suggestions on matings and equine insurance.

Gainesway

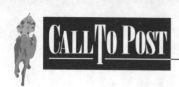

Cookies & Candies

CHOCOLATE MINT SNOW-TOP COOKIES

Combine flour, baking powder and salt. Set aside. Melt 1 cup chocolate chips. Cream butter and sugar together until smooth. Add melted chocolate and vanilla. Add eggs and beat thoroughly. Blend in dry ingredients and remaining ½ cup chocolate chips. Cover dough with plastic wrap and freeze for about 20 minutes or until firm. Shape dough into 1-inch balls, roll in powdered sugar and place on ungreased baking sheet. Bake at 350° for 9 to 10 minutes. Transfer from baking sheet to wire rack for cooling.

Makes 36.

1½ cups all-purpose flour
1½ teaspoons baking powder
¼ teaspoon salt
1 10-ounce package mint chocolate chips, divided
¼ cup plus 2 tablespoons butter, softened
1 cup sugar
1½ teaspoons vanilla
2 eggs
Powdered sugar, sifted

CHOCOLATE CHIP OATMEAL COOKIES

A family favorite!

Cream shortening, sugar and brown sugar together until smooth. Blend in eggs. Combine oats, flour, baking powder, soda and salt. Add dry ingredients to creamed mixture. Stir in chocolate chips. Drop dough by teaspoonfuls on lightly greased baking sheet. Bake at 375° for 10 to 15 minutes or until lightly browned. Transfer from baking sheet to wire rack for cooling.

Makes 60.

1 cup vegetable shortening
¾ cup sugar
¾ cup firmly-packed brown sugar
2 eggs
2 cups rolled oats
2 cups all-purpose flour
½ teaspoon baking powder
1 teaspoon baking soda
½ teaspoon salt
1 teaspoon vanilla
1 6-ounce package semisweet chocolate chips

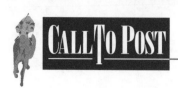

CHUNKY MACADAMIA NUT WHITE CHOCOLATE COOKIES

½ cup butter or margarine, softened
2 tablespoons sugar
¾ cup firmly-packed brown sugar
1 egg
1½ teaspoons vanilla
2 cups all-purpose flour
½ teaspoon baking powder
¾ teaspoon baking soda
⅛ teaspoon salt
1 cup vanilla-milk chips or 1 6-ounce package white chocolate baking bar, cut in chunks
1 7-ounce jar macadamia nuts, coarsely chopped

Using electric mixer, beat butter or margarine until fluffy. Gradually add sugar and brown sugar, beating thoroughly. Add egg and vanilla, mixing well. Combine flour, baking powder, soda and salt. Gradually add dry ingredients to creamed mixture. Add white chocolate and nuts. Drop dough by rounded teaspoonfuls on lightly greased baking sheets. Bake at 350° for 8 to 10 minutes. Transfer from baking sheet to wire rack for cooling.

Makes 60.

OATMEAL CRISPS

½ cup margarine, softened
½ cup sugar
½ cup firmly-packed dark brown sugar
1 egg
1 tablespoon water
1 teaspoon vanilla
1 cup sifted all-purpose flour
½ teaspoon baking powder
½ teaspoon baking soda
¼ teaspoon salt
1½ cups rolled oats
½ cup chopped nuts

Cream margarine, sugar and brown sugar together until smooth. Add egg and beat until fluffy. Sift flour, baking powder, soda and salt together. Add ⅓ of dry ingredients and ½ cup oats to creamed mixture, mixing well. Repeat additions twice, mixing well after each. Fold nuts into dough. Drop dough by teaspoonfuls on greased baking sheet. Bake at 350° for 10 to 12 minutes or until lightly browned. Transfer from baking sheet to wire rack for cooling.

Makes 48 to 60.

KENTUCKY'S BEST COOKIES

Cream butter, sugar and brown sugar together until light and fluffy. Add egg and mix well. Blend in oil and vanilla. Stir in oats, corn flakes, coconut and nuts. Sift flour, baking soda and salt together. Add dry ingredients to oat mixture, mixing well. Drop dough by teaspoonfuls on ungreased baking sheet. Press top of each with fork tines dipped in water. Bake at 325° for 12 minutes. Cool on baking sheet for a few minutes before transferring to wire racks for cooling.

Makes 72.

1 cup butter, softened
1 cup sugar
1 cup firmly-packed brown sugar
1 egg
1 cup vegetable oil
1 teaspoon vanilla
1 cup rolled oats
1 cup crushed corn flakes
1 cup shredded coconut (optional)
½ cup chopped nuts
3½ cups all-purpose flour
1 teaspoon baking soda
1 teaspoon salt

S'MORE COOKIES

Cookies are best when unsalted butter is used.

Cream butter, sugar and brown sugar together until smooth. Blend in egg and vanilla. Combine flour, baking soda and salt. Add dry ingredients to creamed mixture, mixing well. Stir in oats, chocolate chips, raisins and walnuts. Drop dough by tablespoonfuls on greased baking sheet. Bake at 375° for about 10 minutes.

Makes 48.

1 cup unsalted butter, softened
¾ cup sugar
¾ cup firmly packed brown sugar
3 eggs
1 teaspoon vanilla
2 cups all-purpose flour
1 teaspoon baking soda
1 teaspoon salt
1 cup rolled oats
1 12-ounce package semisweet chocolate chips
1 cup raisins
½ cup chopped walnuts

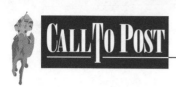

BUTTER NUT SQUARES

½ cup butter, softened
½ cup margarine, softened
1 cup sugar
1 egg, separated
2 cups all-purpose flour
2 teaspoons vanilla
1 cup pecans or almonds,
   broken

Cream butter, margarine and sugar together until smooth. Add egg yolk, flour and vanilla, mixing well. Spread dough thinly on 13x10x1-inch jelly roll pan. Lightly beat egg white. Brush egg white on dough surface and sprinkle with pecans. Bake at 275° for 45 minutes. Transfer from baking sheet to wire rack for cooling. Cut into bars and store in air-tight container.

Makes 48 to 60.

GRAN'S BUTTER COOKIES

1 cup butter, softened
1 cup sugar
1 egg
1 teaspoon vanilla
2 cups all-purpose flour
½ teaspoon baking soda
1 teaspoon salt
   Semisweet chocolate chips or
   colored sugar (optional)

Cream butter and sugar together until smooth. Blend in egg and vanilla. Combine flour, baking soda and salt. Add dry ingredients to creamed mixture, mixing well. Chill dough. Shape dough into small balls, place on ungreased baking sheet and press with fork tines to flatten. Decorate with chocolate chips or colored sugar. Bake at 350° for about 15 minutes or until lightly browned. Transfer from baking sheet to wire rack for cooling.

Makes 96 to 108.

CREAM CHEESE COOKIES

Combine cream cheese and butter, blending until smooth. Combine flour and sugar. Add to creamed mixture, mixing well. Stir in vanilla. Shape dough into small balls and place on ungreased baking sheet. Press chocolate chips or pecans into each ball. Bake at 350° for 12 minutes or until lightly browned. Transfer from baking sheet to wire rack for cooling.

Makes 48 to 60.

1   3-ounce package cream cheese, softened
1   cup butter, softened (do not use margarine)
2   cups all-purpose flour
½   cup sugar
1   tablespoon vanilla
    Semisweet chocolate chips or pecan halves

LACE COOKIES

Combine butter, syrup, brown sugar and oil in saucepan. Bring to a boil, remove from heat and stir in flour and sesame seeds. Let stand for 10 minutes. Drop dough by level tablespoonful 3 inches apart on parchment paper-lined baking sheet (3 cookies per sheet). Bake at 375° for 6 to 7 minutes or until golden brown. Cool on pan for 1 minute or until cookies hold shape when carefully lifted with metal spatula. Place each cookie over inverted custard cup or small bowl. Cool until firm. Allow baking sheet to cool before reusing; parchment paper need not be replaced each time. Spoon fruit filling into cookie shells.

Makes 20.

¼   cup plus 1 tablespoon butter
⅓   cup light corn syrup
½   cup firmly-packed brown sugar
1½ teaspoons sesame oil
¾   cup all-purpose flour
1   tablespoon sesame seeds
1   tablespoon black sesame seeds

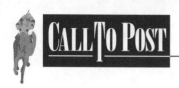

MELT AWAYS
These will disappear in a hurry!

COOKIES
1 cup all-purpose flour
¾ cup cornstarch
½ cup powdered sugar, sifted
1 cup butter, softened

Sift flour, cornstarch and powdered sugar together. Add butter and beat until smooth. Chill dough for 1 hour. Shape into balls and place 1 inch apart on ungreased baking sheet. Bake at 350° for 15 minutes. Transfer from baking sheet to wire rack for cooling. Spread frosting on cooled cookies.

FROSTING
2 tablespoons butter, softened
1 cup powdered sugar, sifted
1 tablespoon lemon extract

Combine butter, sugar and lemon extract. Beat until smooth.

Makes 48.

LEMON SQUARES
A real winner!

CRUST
2 cups all-purpose flour
1 cup powdered sugar, sifted
¼ teaspoon salt
1 cup butter, melted

Combine flour, sugar and salt. Add butter and blend well. Press mixture in bottom of 14x10x2-inch baking pan. Bake at 325° for 20 minutes.

FILLING
¼ cup all-purpose flour
2 cups sugar
¼ cup lemon juice
4 eggs, lightly beaten
Grated peel of 1 lemon
Powdered sugar, sifted

Combine flour, sugar, lemon juice, eggs and lemon peel, mixing well. Pour over baked crust. Bake at 325° for additional 25 minutes. Cool in pan. Sprinkle with powdered sugar and cut in 1½-inch squares. Store in refrigerator.

Makes 54.

PECAN CHEWIES

Combine margarine, brown sugar, eggs and vanilla, beating until smooth. Combine flour, baking powder and salt. Add dry ingredients to egg mixture. Spread batter in greased and floured 13x9x2-inch baking dish. Bake at 350° for 20 to 25 minutes and center is firm; do not overbake. Sprinkle pecans on baked surface, pressing gently. Let stand until cool, then sprinkle with powdered sugar. Cut into 2-inch squares.

Makes 24.

½ cup margarine, softened
1½ cups firmly-packed brown sugar
2 eggs
2 teaspoons vanilla
1½ cups all-purpose flour
1 teaspoon baking powder
¼ teaspoon salt
½ cup chopped pecans
1 tablespoon powdered sugar

BEST BROWNIES
No one can eat just one!

Combine eggs, sugar and vanilla, beating thoroughly. Blend in butter. Combine flour, cocoa and salt. Add dry ingredients to egg mixture, mixing well. Stir in nuts. Pour batter into 15x10x2-inch glass baking dish. Bake at 350° for 35 minutes. Cool in pan. Spread frosting on cooled brownies and cut into 2-inch squares.

Combine butter, honey, vanilla and milk. Using electric mixer, blend powered sugar and cocoa, mixing until smooth.

Makes 35.

BROWNIES
8 eggs, beaten
4 cups sugar
2 teaspoons vanilla
2 cups butter, melted
2 cups all-purpose flour
1 cup cocoa
1 teaspoon salt
2 cups chopped nuts

FROSTING
¼ cup plus 2 tablespoons butter, softened
2 tablespoons honey
1 teaspoon vanilla
2 to 4 tablespoons milk
2 cups powdered sugar, sifted
¼ cup plus 2 tablespoons cocoa

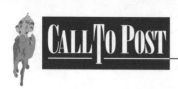
CHOCOLATE SWIRL BROWNIES

BROWNIES
1 6-ounce package semisweet chocolate chips
¼ cup plus 2 tablespoons butter
½ cup sugar
2 eggs
1 teaspoon vanilla
½ cup all-purpose flour
½ teaspoon baking powder

Melt chocolate and butter together in large saucepan over low heat. Remove from heat, add sugar and mix well. Blend in eggs and vanilla. Sift flour and baking powder together. Add dry ingredients to chocolate mixture. Pour ½ of batter into greased and floured 9x9x2-inch baking pan. Bake at 350° for 10 minutes. Prepare filling as directed. Pour filling over baked layer, spoon remaining chocolate mixture on cheese filling and swirl with knife tip. Bake at 350° for additional 35 to 45 minutes. Cool in pan. Cut into 2-inch squares.

CREAM CHEESE FILLING
1 8-ounce package cream cheese, softened
½ cup sugar
   Dash of salt
1 egg
½ cup chopped pecans

Combine cream cheese, sugar and salt, beating until smooth. Fold egg into mixture. Stir in pecans.

Makes 16.

CHOCOLATE CHIP CREAM PUFFS

½ cup water
¼ cup unsalted butter
½ cup all-purpose flour
2 eggs
1 tablespoon finely chopped semisweet chocolate

Combine water and butter in saucepan and bring to a boil. Add flour and blend until smooth. Reduce heat and cook for 2 minutes. Place batter in mixing bowl. Using electric mixer, beat in eggs, 1 at a time. Let stand until cooled to room temperature. Stir in chocolate pieces. Drop by tablespoonfuls on parchment paper-lined baking sheet. Bake at 400° for 30 to 35 minutes or until puffs are golden brown and firm to touch. Store in covered container after puffs are cooled.

Makes 6.

BOURBON BALLS

Combine milk, bourbon, butter, powdered sugar and pecans, mixing thoroughly. Chill for 1 hour. Shape mixture into balls and place on small baking sheet. Chill until firm. Melt semisweet and unsweetened chocolate with paraffin in top of double boiler over very hot water. Using wooden pick, dip bourbon balls in liquid chocolate and place on wax paper on baking sheet. Chill until coating is firm. Store in refrigerator.

Makes 150.

½ cup sweetened condensed milk
1 cup 100 proof bourbon
2⅔ tablespoons butter
3 16-ounce packages powdered sugar, sifted
1 cup chopped pecans
½ pound semisweet chocolate
½ pound unsweetened chocolate
⅓ bar (4x2-inch) paraffin

ENGLISH TOFFEE

Sprinkle 1 cup pecans on rimmed baking sheet. Sprinkle 1 cup chocolate on pecans. Combine sugar, butter and water in heavy saucepan over medium heat. Cook until syrup reaches 290° on candy thermometer. Remove from heat and blend in vanilla. Pour over chocolate layer, quickly sprinkle with remaining 1 cup chocolate and top with remaining 1 cup nuts. Using wax paper, press gently on layers. Let stand until cool and dry. Break into pieces.

Makes about 1½ pounds.

2 cups grated sweet chocolate, divided
2 cups chopped pecans, divided
1 cup raw sugar
1 cup butter
1 tablespoon water
1 teaspoon vanilla

CHOW MEIN CANDY
Easy and fun for kids to make.

Combine frosting, noodles, marshmallows, pecans and vanilla, mixing well. Drop by tablespoonfuls on wax paper. Let stand until firm.

Makes 2 dozen.

1 16-ounce can milk chocolate frosting
½ cup chow mein noodles
½ cup miniature marshmallows
½ cup chopped pecans
1 teaspoon vanilla

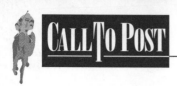

CHOCOLATE TURTLES

1 6-ounce package semisweet
  chocolate chips
1 3½-ounce jar marshmallow
  creme
1 cup pecan halves
2¼ cups sugar
½ 13-ounce can evaporated milk
¼ cup margarine

Combine chocolate chips, marshmallow creme and pecans, stirring gently but not mixing. Combine sugar, evaporated milk and margarine in a saucepan. Cook, stirring constantly, over low heat, until mixture comes to a boil. Cook for 7½ minutes. Remove from heat, pour over chocolate mixture and mix well. Drop by heaping teaspoonfuls on wax paper. Let stand until firm.

Makes 55.

BUCKEYES

3 16-ounce packages powdered
  sugar, sifted
2 16-ounce jars creamy peanut
  butter
2 cups margarine, melted
½ bar (4x2 inch) paraffin
2 12-ounce packages semisweet
  chocolate chips

Combine powdered sugar, peanut butter and margarine, mixing by hand until smooth. Shape into bite-sized balls. Combine paraffin and chocolate chips in top of double boiler over very hot water, stirring until melted and blended. Using wooden pick, dip peanut butter balls into chocolate, covering about ⅔ of surface, and place on wax paper on baking sheet. Chill until firm.

Makes 200.

CARAMELS

5 cups sugar
2 cups light corn syrup
4 cups whipping cream,
  divided
1 teaspoon vanilla

Combine sugar, syrup and 2 cups cream in saucepan. Bring to a boil. Stirring constantly, gradually add remaining 2 cups cream; mixture should continue boiling. Cook for about 1½ hours or until mixture reaches 250° on candy thermometer. Remove from heat and add vanilla. Pour into large buttered pan. Let stand until cool, cut into squares and wrap in plastic wrap squares.

Makes 250.

Desserts

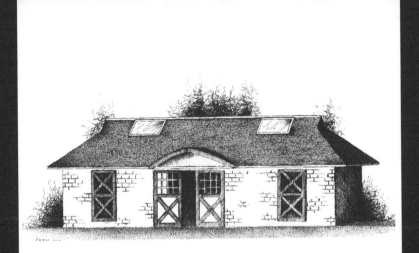

Just as gourmet food requires premium ingredients and the skill to prepare it, a racehorse results from many factors. A runner must have the proper genetics, a good attitude, sound build and appropriate handling to become a top performer. At Taylor Made Farm, our skilled team members work daily to prepare the ingredients of a potential racehorse. Located in Nicholasville, Kentucky, Taylor Made is a public sales agency, nursery, and stands the stallions Unbridled's Song and Candy Stripes. Over the years, Taylor Made has prepared champions Dancing Brave, Dayjur and Manila, as well as Grade I winners Devil His Due, Louis Quatorze, Maplejinsky, November Snow, Tiffany Lass, Twist Afleet, West by West, Classy Mirage, Unbridled's Song, etc.

Taylor Made

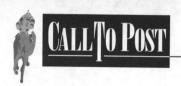

Desserts

APPLE CRISP

Combine apples, ½ cup sugar, ½ cup brown sugar, pinch of salt, cinnamon, nutmeg and rum, tossing to coat evenly. Spread mixture in heavily buttered 13x9x2-inch baking dish. Using pastry blender or 2 table knives, cut flour and butter together. Add remaining ½ cup sugar, ½ cup brown sugar, pinch of salt and walnuts or pecans, tossing to combine. Spread topping in thick layer over apples. Bake at 350° for about 45 minutes or until the top is nicely browned and the apples are syrupy. Serve with whipped cream.

Serves 6 to 8.

10 medium Granny Smith apples, peeled, cored and thinly sliced
1 cup sugar, divided
1 cup firmly-packed brown sugar, divided
Pinch of salt
1 tablespoon cinnamon
1 teaspoon nutmeg
2 tablespoons dark rum
1½ cups all-purpose flour
1 cup unsalted butter
1½ cups broken walnuts or pecans
Sweetened whipped cream (optional)

GINGERBREAD

A tradition!

Combine molasses, sugar, margarine, cloves or allspice and ginger. Dissolve soda in boiling water and add to molasses mixture. Blend in flour and eggs. Batter will be very thin. Pour into greased and floured 9x9x2-inch baking pan. Bake at 375° for 30 minutes. Cool in pan. Cut in squares and serve with lemon sauce. Store in covered container.

Pour water into saucepan and bring to a boil. Blend in sugar and flour. Bring to a boil and cook for several minutes. Stir in lemon juice and peel. Cook until slightly thickened, remove from heat and stir in butter.

Serves 9.

BREAD
1 cup molasses
½ cup sugar
½ cup margarine, melted
2 teaspoons ground cloves or allspice
2 teaspoons ginger
½ teaspoon soda
1 cup boiling water
2½ cups sifted all-purpose flour
2 eggs, well beaten

SAUCE
1 cup boiling water
1 cup sugar
1 tablespoon all-purpose flour
Juice and grated peel of 1 lemon
2 tablespoons butter

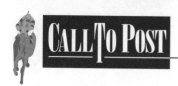

FRUIT COBBLER

FILLING
- 6 cups fresh or frozen fruit
- 2½ cups sugar

PASTRY
- 2 cups all-purpose flour
- 1 tablespoon sugar
- 1 teaspoon salt
- ¾ cup vegetable shortening
- ⅓ to ½ cup ice water
- ½ cup butter, melted
- ½ to ¾ cup sugar

Combine fruit and sugar. Let stand for a day or overnight to allow formation of juices.

Combine flour, 1 tablespoon sugar and salt. Using pastry blender or 2 table knives, cut vegetable into dry ingredients. Gradually add water, working with fingers, until dough forms a ball. Divide dough in 2 portions. On lightly floured surface, roll ½ of dough into rectangle to cover bottom and sides of 13x9x2-inch baking pan. Pour fruit and juice into pastry-lined pan. Roll remaining dough to rectangle shape to fit over fruit and to edges of pan; do not seal. Prick top pastry with fork tines to vent steam. Drizzle butter over pastry and sprinkle with ½ to ¾ cup sugar. Bake at 425° for 45 minutes or until golden brown and juices are bubbly. Cool in pan.

Serves 8.

FRUIT TORTE

- ½ cup butter, softened
- 1 cup sugar
- 1 cup all-purpose flour
- 1 teaspoon baking powder
- ¼ teaspoon salt
- 2 eggs
- 2 cups blueberries, raspberries, strawberries, peaches or other fruit of your choice
  Sugar
  Lemon juice
  Cinnamon

Cream butter and sugar together until smooth. Combine flour, baking powder and salt. Add dry ingredients and eggs to creamed mixture. Spread batter in 9-inch spring form pan. Spoon fruit on batter and sprinkle generously with sugar, lemon juice and cinnamon. Bake at 350° for 1 hour. Cool in pan, release sides and serve.

Serves 8.

RED RASPBERRY TART

Combine flour and sugar. Using pastry blender or 2 table knives, cut butter into dry ingredients until texture of coarse meal. Blend in cold water. Press pastry into tart pan or in bottom and 1 inch along sides of spring form pan. Prick pastry with fork tines. Bake at 350° for 25 minutes or until browned.

PASTRY
- 1¼ cups all-purpose flour
- ¼ cup sugar
- ½ cup butter
- 2 tablespoons cold water

While crust is baking, combine cream cheese, sugar, vanilla and egg, beating until smooth. Blend in flour. Pour filling into baked crust. Bake at 350° for 20 to 25 minutes. Cool in pan. Combine jam and lemon juice in saucepan. Heat until jam is melted and mixture is smooth. Arrange raspberries on cooled tart and brush with warm jam.

Serves 8.

FILLING
- 1 8-ounce package cream cheese, softened
- ½ cup sugar
- 1 teaspoon vanilla
- 1 egg, beaten
    tablespoon all-purpose flour
- ¼ cup raspberry jam
- 1 tablespoon lemon juice
- 3 cups fresh raspberries

TIRAMISU
Elegant!

Combine egg yolks, sugar and wine in top of double boiler. Cook over hot water until sugar is dissolved. Remove from heat and continue stirring until cool. Combine mascarpone cream and whipping cream, beating until smooth. Blend into custard. Lightly soak lady fingers in espresso. Place a single layer of lady fingers in 12x8x2-inch baking dish. Sprinkle with 1 tablespoon cocoa and spoon ½ custard on lady fingers. Repeat layers and top with chocolate shavings. Chill for at least 2 hours.

Serves 8.

- 4 egg yolks
- 1¼ cups sugar
- ¼ cup Marsala wine
- 1 cup mascarpone cream
- 1 cup whipping cream
- 30 lady fingers
- 6 cups espresso, at room temperature
- 2 tablespoons cocoa
- 2 1-ounce squares semisweet chocolate, shaved

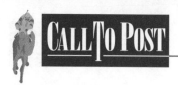

CHEESECAKE

PASTRY
¼ cup plus 2 tablespoons butter or margarine, melted
2½ cups graham cracker crumbs
½ cup sugar

Combine butter or margarine, crumbs and sugar, mixing until evenly moist. Prepare a 10-inch spring form pan with vegetable cooking spray. Sprinkle crumbs along sides to ¾ of pan depth; reserving ¼ cup crumbs, press remainder in bottom of pan, tightly sealing around edge.

FILLING
6 eggs, separated
1½ cups sugar, divided
3 8-ounce packages cream cheese, softened
½ cup all-purpose flour
1½ cups sour cream
1½ tablespoons lemon juice
1 tablespoon vanilla

Using electric mixer, beat egg yolks, ¾ cup sugar, cream cheese, flour, sour cream, lemon juice and vanilla together until very smooth and creamy. Clean mixer beaters and in separate bowl, beat egg whites until frothy. Add remaining ¾ cup sugar and beat until stiff peaks form. Fold egg whites into cream mixture, mixing gently. Spread filling in prepared spring form pan and sprinkle reserved ¼ cup crumbs over surface. Bake at 325° for 1 hour, turn oven off but do not open oven door for 1 additional hour. Cool cheesecake to room temperature before storing in refrigerator. **Note:** Serve cheesecake wedge with fresh sliced unsweetened strawberries or with fruit topping.

Serves 10.

BUTTERSCOTCH BOMBE

Combine crumbs and melted butter. Press crumbs in 10-inch spring form pan. Freeze until firm. Slightly soften ice cream and stir in crushed candy. Spoon ice cream into prepared crust, pressing firmly, and refreeze.

Combine brown sugar, half and half and butter in saucepan. Cook over low heat until blended and warm. Stir in vanilla and almonds. Release sides of spring form pan. Cut slices, place on individual plates and spoon sauce over ice cream.

Serves 6 to 8.

BOMBE

1½ cups crushed ginger snaps
3 tablespoons butter, melted
½ gallon coffee ice cream
6 chocolate toffee candy bars, crushed

SAUCE

1 cup firmly-packed brown sugar
1 cup half and half
½ cup butter
1 teaspoon vanilla
½ cup sliced almonds, toasted

LIGHT CARAMEL KAHLÚA SQUARES

Combine crumbs and margarine, mixing well. Sprinkle ½ of crumbs in 8x8x2-inch baking pan prepared with vegetable cooking spray. Stir Kahlúa into ice cream. Spread ½ of ice cream on crumb crust. Combine syrup and coffee. Drizzle ½ of caramel mixture over ice cream. Freeze until firm. Repeat layers with remaining ice cream and caramel mixture and sprinkle with remaining crumbs. Freeze until firm.

Serves 9.

¼ cup plus 1 tablespoon chocolate wafer crumbs
2 teaspoons low-fat margarine, melted
2 tablespoons Kahlúa or other coffee-flavored liqueur
6 cups low-fat vanilla ice cream, softened
½ cup fat-free caramel flavored syrup
2 tablespoons strongly brewed coffee

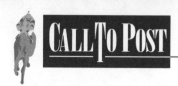

COFFEE ICE CREAM

3 tablespoons instant coffee
   granules
1 cup milk
1 cup sugar
1½ teaspoons vanilla
4½ cups whipping cream

Combine coffee, milk, sugar and vanilla in blender or food processor, mixing until sugar is dissolved. Pour into stainless steel bowl. Whisk in cream. Chill thoroughly, then freeze in ice cream freezer following manufacturer's directions. **Note:** About ⅓ cup coffee-flavored liqueur can be added; reduce whipping cream by ⅓ cup.

Makes about 3 quarts.

PEPPERMINT ICE CREAM

½ pound red-striped
   peppermint stick candy,
   crushed
2 cups half and half
2 cups whipping cream
⅛ teaspoon salt

Soak candy in half and half overnight. If not dissolved, heat slightly to melt, then cool. Combine whipping cream with peppermint cream and salt. Freeze in ice cream freezer following manufacturer's directions.

Serves 6 to 8.

HIGH HAMPTON BUTTERSCOTCH SAUCE

Fabulous sauce on vanilla ice cream.

½ cup firmly-packed light
   brown sugar
⅓ cup light corn syrup
2 tablespoons butter
⅛ teaspoon salt
½ cup whipping cream

Combine brown sugar, syrup, butter and salt in heavy saucepan. Bring to a boil, reduce heat and cook, stirring constantly, until mixture reaches soft ball stage (234° on candy thermometer). Remove from heat and let stand for 5 minutes. Blend in whipping cream.

Makes 1 cup.

PRESERVES, PICKLES & RELISHES

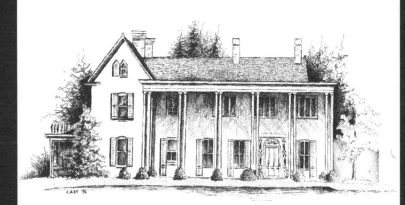

Located just outside Lexington along Paris Pike, Walmac International is a full-service facility which stands twenty-four stallions, offers boarding and breaking and training, as well as sale preparation and representation. Their impressive stallion roster includes proven stallions Alleged, Miswaki and Nureyev, as well as promising young hopefuls Salt Lake, Talkin Man and West by West.

Walmac

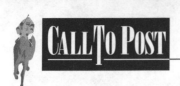

Preserves, Pickles & Relishes

CANNING

Always use clean jars. Wash jars well before you begin so that when your canning mixture is ready, your jars are also. With jams and jellies, contaminants which could cause spoilage are destroyed when the hot canning mixtures are poured into jars and immediately covered and inverted for 5 minutes to seal the cooked jam or jelly. Other canning recipes may need the traditional method of boiling jars in water to sterilize.

GRAPE JELLY

3½	pounds ripe Concord grapes
½	cup water
7	cups sugar
½	1¾-ounce packet fruit pectin

Sort, wash and remove stems from grapes. Crush grapes. Combine pulp and water in heavy saucepan. Cover and bring to a boil over high heat, reduce heat and simmer for 10 minutes. Extract juice from pulp. To avoid formation of tartrate crystals in jelly, let stand in cool place overnight. Strain through 2 thicknesses cheesecloth to remove crystals. Combine 4 cups juice and sugar in large heavy saucepan or kettle. Place over high heat and, stirring constantly, quickly bring to a full rolling boil which cannot be stirred down. Add pectin, bring to a boil and cook for 1 minute. Remove from heat and quickly skim foam. Immediately pour jelly into hot sterilized 8-ounce jars and seal according to manufacturer's directions.

Makes 8 or 9.

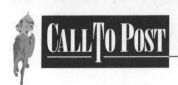

BLACKBERRY JAM

2 quarts ripe blackberries
7 cups sugar
½ 1¾-ounce packet fruit pectin

Crush berries, 1 layer at a time. If desired, press ½ of pulp through sieve to remove some of seeds. Combine 4 cups pulp and sugar in large saucepan, mixing well. Bring to a full boil over high heat and cook for 1 minute, stirring constantly. Remove from heat and stir in pectin. Skim foam from surface with metal spoon. Stir, continuing to skim foam, for 5 minutes to slightly cool mixture and prevent floating fruit. Ladle jam into hot sterilized 6-ounce jars and seal with lids according to manufacturer's directions.

Makes 10.

FRESH PEACH JAM

3 pounds ripe peaches
  Boiling water
¼ cup lemon juice (optional)
7½ cups sugar
1 1¾-ounce packet fruit pectin

Dip peaches, a few at a time, into boiling water to release skins, then into cold water. Remove skins, split and remove pits. Grind or finely chop peaches. Combine 4 cups pulp, lemon juice if sharper flavor desired, and sugar in large saucepan, mixing well. Place over high heat and, stirring constantly, bring to a full rolling boil and cook for 1 minute. Remove from heat and immediately stir in pectin. Stir, skimming foam as it forms, for 5 minutes. Ladle jam into hot sterilized 6-ounce jars and seal with lids according to manufacturer's directions.

Makes 11.

STRAWBERRY JAM

Crush fruit, 1 layer at a time. Combine 4½ cups pulp and pectin in very large saucepan. Place over high heat and bring to a hard boil, stirring constantly. Immediately stir in sugar. Bring to a full rolling boil and cook hard for 1 minute, stirring constantly. Remove from heat and skim foam with metal spoon. Stir, continuing to skim foam, for 5 minutes to slightly cool and to prevent floating fruit. Ladle into hot sterilized 8-ounce jars and seal with lids according to manufacturer's directions.

Makes 11.

2 **quarts ripe strawberries, stems removed**
1 **1¾-ounce packet fruit pectin**
7 **cups sugar**

FRESH STRAWBERRY JELLY

Crush strawberries by placing in jelly bag and squeezing to produce 3½ cups juice; if insufficient, add small amount of water to pulp and squeeze again. Combine juice and pectin in heavy saucepan. Bring to a rapid boil, add salt and sugar and cook for 1 minute, stirring constantly. Remove from heat and skim foam. Immediately ladle into hot sterilized 8-ounce jars, leaving ½-inch headspace. Seal according to manufacturer's directions.

Makes 6.

2½ **quarts fresh strawberries, stems removed**
1 **1¾-ounce packet fruit pectin**
¼ **teaspoon salt**
5 **cups sugar**

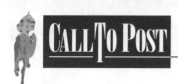

SPICED PEACHES

4   pounds peaches
    Salted water
1   tablespoon whole allspice
2   teaspoons whole cloves
2   3-inch cinnamon sticks
4½ cups sugar
1½ cups cider vinegar
¾   cup water

Peel peaches, placing in slightly salted water to prevent discoloring. Place allspice, cloves and cinnamon sticks in cheesecloth bag. Combine sugar, vinegar, ¾ cup water and spice bag in 5-quart kettle. Bring to a boil, add peaches, return to boil, reduce heat and simmer for 10 minutes or until tender. Place in large bowl. Chill, covered, overnight. Discard spice bag. Spoon peaches into sterilized 1-pint jars. Pour syrup over peaches, leaving ½ inch headspace. Place lids on jars and process in boiling water bath according to jar manufacturer's directions.

Makes 4.

PEAR CHUTNEY

½   pound onions, sliced
4   pounds pears, cored and cut
    in chunks
2   pounds Sultana raisins
2   pounds candied dried ginger
¼   cup chopped garlic
6½ cups sugar
¼   cup salt
1¼ teaspoons cayenne pepper
½   teaspoon cinnamon
½   teaspoon ground cloves
1½ teaspoons ground ginger
¼   teaspoon mace
1½ teaspoons paprika
3   quarts dark cider vinegar

Combine onions, pears, raisins, ginger and garlic in stock pot. Add sugar, salt, cayenne pepper, cinnamon, cloves, ginger, mace and paprika. Stir in vinegar. Simmer for 3 hours. Ladle chutney into hot sterilized 1-pint jars and seal according to manufacturer's directions.

Makes 12.

CORN RELISH

Combine corn, cabbage, onion, green bell pepper, red bell pepper and bay leaf in stock pot. Add vinegar, sugar, water, pickling salt, celery seed, mustard seed and turmeric. Place over medium-high heat and bring to a boil, stirring occasionally. Reduce heat to medium and cook for 15 minutes, stirring occasionally. Remove bay leaf. Immediately ladle into hot sterilized 1-pint jars, leaving ½-inch headspace and stirring with plastic spoon to remove air bubbles. Place hot lids on jars, seal and process in boiling water canner for 15 minutes.

Makes 5 or 6.

6	cups fresh whole kernel corn (about 12 ears), cooked
3	cups chopped cabbage
1	cup chopped onion
1	medium green bell pepper, chopped
1	medium red bell pepper, chopped
1	bay leaf
4	cups white vinegar
2	cups sugar
1	cup water
1	tablespoon pickling salt
1	tablespoon celery seed
1	tablespoon mustard seed
1	tablespoon turmeric

QUICK CHOW-CHOW

Combine cabbage, tomatoes, onion, green bell peppers and red bell peppers. Layer in enamel pan or stone jar, sprinkling each layer well with salt and covering top layer with salt. Let stand overnight. Drain well the following morning. Combine vinegar, sugar, mustard, celery seed, mustard seed and cloves (in cheesecloth bag) in stock pot. Bring to a boil. Add well-drained vegetables and cook over medium-low heat for about 30 minutes or until tender. Discard cloves bag. Pack chow-chow in hot sterilized 1-pint jars. Place hot lids on jars, seal and process in hot water bath for 10 minutes at simmering temperature.

Makes 8 to 10.

4	cups chopped cabbage
2	cups chopped green tomatoes
3	onions, chopped
1½	green bell peppers, chopped
1½	red bell peppers, chopped
1	cup salt
4	cups vinegar
2	cups sugar
2	tablespoons dry mustard
2¼	teaspoons celery seed
1½	tablespoons white mustard seed
1	teaspoon whole cloves

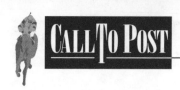

SWEET GREEN TOMATO RELISH

2 gallons small green tomatoes, chopped
1 head cabbage, chopped
3 potatoes, diced
6 onions, diced
6 apples, cored and diced
3 green bell peppers, chopped
3 red bell peppers, chopped
Coarse salt
2 cups sugar
1 cup firmly-packed brown sugar
Vinegar

Place tomatoes, cabbage, potatoes, onion, apples, green bell peppers and red bell peppers in sack. Sprinkle handful of coarse salt on top of vegetables. Let drain overnight. Drain well the following morning. Combine vegetables, sugar and brown sugar in stock pot. Add vinegar to cover and simmer for 30 minutes. Add sugar if sweeter flavor preferred. Ladle relish into hot sterilized 1-pint jars. Place hot lids on jars, seal and process according to manufacturer's directions.

Makes 8.

VEGETABLE RELISH

2½ pounds cucumbers, peeled and cut in ½-inch pieces
2 large white onions, cut in ½-inch chunks
2 large green bell peppers, seeded and cut in ½-inch chunks
1 small head cauliflower, cut in ½-inch chunks
½ pound carrots, shredded
½ pound celery, cut in ½-inch pieces
½ cup pickling salt
1 bag ice
4 cups cider vinegar
4 cups sugar
2 teaspoons celery seed
1 tablespoon plus 1 teaspoon mustard seed
2 teaspoons red pepper flakes
2 teaspoons ground turmeric

Combine cucumbers, onion, bell pepper, cauliflower, carrots and celery in stock pot. Cover with salt. Pour ice on vegetables to cover. Let stand for 24 hours, adding ice as needed. Rinse vegetables and drain well. Bring to a boil, stirring constantly. Ladle relish in hot sterilized 1-pint jars. Cover with lids. Store in refrigerator for 3 weeks before serving.

Makes 8.

CHICAGO HOT SAUCE

Drain tomato slices overnight. Combine slices, onion, celery, horseradish, hot pepper sauce, green bell peppers, red bell peppers, mustard seeds, sugar and salt in stock pot. Add vinegar, mixing well. Bring to a boil. Ladle sauce into hot sterilized 1-pint jars. Place hot lids on jars, seal and process according to manufacturer's directions.

Makes 8.

2 gallons ripe tomato slices
2 cups chopped onion
2 cups chopped celery
1 cup grated horseradish
1 cup hot pepper sauce
2 green bell peppers, chopped
2 red bell peppers, chopped
½ cup mustard seed
2 cups sugar
½ cup salt
6 cups vinegar

CUCUMBER LIME PICKLES

Soak cucumbers in mixture of lime and water in crockery or enamel container for 12 hours or overnight; do not use aluminum container. Drain and discard lime water. Rinse cucumbers 3 times in fresh cold water, then soak in fresh ice water for 3 hours. Combine vinegar, sugar, salt and pickling spices in stock pot. Bring to a low boil, stirring until sugar is dissolved. Remove from heat and add cucumbers. Let stand for 5 to 6 hours or overnight. Bring to a boil and cook for 35 minutes. Ladle cucumbers into hot sterilized 1-pint jars. Add hot syrup, leaving ½-inch headspace. Place hot lids on jars, seal and process in boiling water bath canner for 10 minutes. Store unsealed jars in refrigerator.

Makes 8.

7 pounds cucumbers, sliced
1 cup pickling lime
2 gallons water
8 cups distilled white vinegar (5% acidity)
8 cups sugar
1 tablespoon salt (optional)
2 teaspoons mixed pickling spices

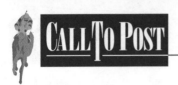

BEAUTIFUL BREAD AND BUTTER PICKLES

3 quarts sliced cucumbers
3 large onions, sliced
½ cup salt
Water
3 cups vinegar
3 cups firmly-packed brown sugar
1½ teaspoons celery seed
1 teaspoon cinnamon
½ teaspoon ground ginger
2 tablespoons mustard seed
1 teaspoon ground turmeric
1 hot pepper or 1 tablespoon grated horseradish (optional)

Combine cucumbers, onion and salt in large bowl of water. Let stand for 5 hours. Drain well. Combine vinegar, 1 cup water, brown sugar, celery seed, cinnamon, ginger, mustard seed, turmeric and hot pepper or horseradish in stock pot. Bring to a boil and cook for 3 minutes. Add vegetables. Simmer for 10 to 20 minutes; do not boil. Ladle pickles into hot sterilized 1-pint jars. Place hot lids on jars, seal and process in boiling water bath for 5 minutes.

Makes 8.

ICED GREEN TOMATO PICKLE

7 pounds green tomatoes, sliced
3 cups powdered pickling lime
2 gallons water
10 cups sugar
1 gallon vinegar
1 teaspoon allspice
1 teaspoon celery seed
1 teaspoon cinnamon
1 teaspoon cloves
1 teaspoon ginger
1 teaspoon mace
Green food coloring (optional)

Soak tomato slices in mixture of lime and water in crockery or enamel container for 24 hours. Drain and discard lime water. Soak tomatoes in fresh water for 4 hours, changing water at 30 minute intervals. Drain well to assure complete removal of lime. Combine sugar, vinegar, allspice, celery seed, cinnamon, cloves, ginger and mace in stock pot. Bring to a boil, add green food coloring and pour over tomatoes. Let stand overnight. Cook for 1 hour or until tomatoes are translucent. Ladle into hot sterilized 1-pint jars. Place hot lids on jars and seal according to manufacturer's directions.

Makes 7.

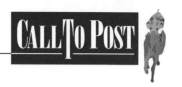

❧ EQUIVALENT MEASURES AND WEIGHTS ❧

Dash	= ¹⁄₁₆ teaspoon or half of ⅛ teaspoon
3 teaspoons	= 1 tablespoon
2 tablespoons	= ⅛ cup or 1 fluid ounce
4 tablespoons	= ¼ cup
5 ⅓ tablespoons	= ⅓ cup
8 tablespoons	= ½ cup
12 tablespoons	= ¾ cup
16 tablespoons	= 1 cup
1 cup	= 8 fluid ounces
2 cups	= 1 pint or 16 fluid ounces
4 cups	= 2 pints or 1 quart or 32 fluid ounces
4 quarts	= 1 gallon
8 quarts	= 1 peck
4 pecks	= 1 bushel
16 ounces	= 1 pound
1 ounce	= 28.35 grams
1 liter	= 1.06 quarts

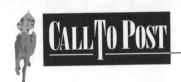
⇥ MEASURING EQUIPMENT ⇤

- *Liquid Measures.* Liquid measuring cups tend to be glass, come in 1-, 2- and 4-cup sizes and have graded measurements indicated on the surface. To measure liquids, place the cup on a level surface and fill, reading the measuring mark at eye level.

- *Dry Measures.* Dry measuring cups come in nested sets that can include ¼-cup, ⅓-cup, ½-cup and 1-cup measures. They are meant to be filled to the top and leveled off with a knife.

- *Shortening and Brown Sugar.* To measure shortening and brown sugar, firmly press into a dry measuring cup and level off with a spatula or knife.

- *Dry ingredients.* To measure flour, sugar and other dry ingredients, lightly spoon the ingredient into the measuring cup and then level it off with the straight edge of a spatula or knife. Flour does not need additional sifting.

Index

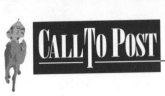

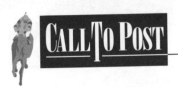

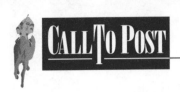

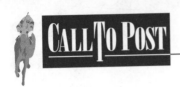

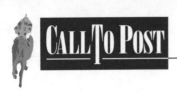

CALL TO POST

635 Iron Works Pike
Lexington, Kentucky 40511
(606) 293-6579

Please send _____ copies   @ $18.95 each _____

Kentucky residents add sales tax   @ $1.14 each _____

Postage and handling   @ $3.50 per order _____ **3.50** _____

                                     Total _____

Name _____

Address _____

City _____ State _____ Zip _____

Make checks payable to *CALL TO POST*

CALL TO POST

635 Iron Works Pike
Lexington, Kentucky 40511
(606) 293-6579

Please send _____ copies   @ $18.95 each _____

Kentucky residents add sales tax   @ $1.14 each _____

Postage and handling   @ $3.50 per order _____ **3.50** _____

                                     Total _____

Name _____

Address _____

City _____ State _____ Zip _____

Make checks payable to *CALL TO POST*

CALL TO POST

635 Iron Works Pike
Lexington, Kentucky 40511
(606) 293-6579

Please send _____ copies   @ $18.95 each _____

Kentucky residents add sales tax   @ $1.14 each _____

Postage and handling   @ $3.50 per order _____ **3.50** _____

                                     Total _____

Name _____

Address _____

City _____ State _____ Zip _____

Make checks payable to *CALL TO POST*